CORONAVIRUS
(COVID-19)
OUTBREAK & THE LOST TREASURE

AuthorHouse™ UK
1663 Liberty Drive
Bloomington, IN 47403   USA
www.authorhouse.co.uk
Phone: 0800 047 8203 (Domestic TFN)
+44 1908 723714 (International)

Because of the dynamic nature of the Internet, any web addresses or links contained in this book may have changed
since publication and may no longer be valid. The views expressed in this work are solely those of the author and do not
necessarily reflect the views of the publisher, and the publisher hereby disclaims any responsibility for them.

This book is printed on acid-free paper.

ISBN: 978-1-7283-5242-8 (sc)
ISBN: 978-1-7283-5241-1 (e)

Print information available on the last page.

Published by AuthorHouse 04/24/2020

authorHOUSE®

CORONAVIRUS (COVID-19)

OUTBREAK & THE LOST TREASURE

FARIS ALHAJRI - PH.D.(A.M.)

INSCRIPTION

One secret to achieving complete and comprehensive holistic health in all PEMS—physical, emotional, mental, spiritual—aspects of life is the moment a human being fully acknowledges, esteems, honors, and embraces all aspects of humanity in respect to gender, race, culture, religion, creed, etc.

This is encouraged immensely by reinfusing the body with the *Four Essential Elements of Life (FEEL)*. These natural elements are necessary for the first step in the life cycle of a zygote. From the formation, reproduction, and division of cells to complete fetal growth, these elements make life on Earth possible.

We are delighted to dedicate the research and findings in this book and in following manuscripts to the people of the world without any limitations. Our passion is to share this sacred universal solvent *"Haqua"* (hot aqua), otherwise publicly known as hot water, while acknowledging and paying tribute to every human's value. Regardless of belief or nationality, we are devoted to the Universal Laws of Nature in which we are all united. We simply care that YOU ARE A HUMAN BEING who possess three common factors: devotion, physical body, and dreams/ambitions.

We deeply believe that real and sustainable success takes place from the inside out, and so we must pay the highest tribute to those loved ones who make this all possible.

I am blessed to be surrounded by a beautiful family: my lovely angel and wife, Gloria, and two beloved sons, Qais and Sami, who are my best friends.

Thank you, my beautiful wife Gloria, for standing with me in all challenges we went through resembling the "Valleys of Death," but you always encouraged me to keep moving forward with my childhood dream.

Thank you to my son Qais for all of your support, and for your advice in proposing the word "Haqua" while filing our trademark.

Thank you to my son Sami for your advice, including the most prominent, where I learned from you these two most crucial lessons: "Start small and grow big;" "To deal with People is like a door that needs the right Key."

I am blessed by this family's full emotional support as I pursue my advocacy, and most importantly, for encouraging me in their full implementation of the BICADU Principles—believe, implement, continue, appreciate, discipline, and understand.

I love every person who believes in enhancing health, peace, tenderness, coherence, and cultural competence. Though I am not able to meet in person each of these amazing individuals, my soul is with each one of them. Somewhere, somehow, we shall meet.

I shifted into the Universal Laws of Nature, the Universal Faith that unites us all, without the fear of mankind. I pay my highest tribute to all people, while keeping loyal to where I came from and where I am going.

I choose love and acceptance, not hate, and avoid all who induce hatred or who commit atrocities against others.

I may not know you when we meet. I may not understand your unique personality or appreciate all that you have gone through in this journey called Life. Nonetheless, a platonic love connects us all. No matter your physical or financial potential, culture, race, or religion, we are all descendants of one family. You are my family.

At times I may fear the future, but I choose to focus on the truths of *Climbing the Endless Mountains of Life (CEML)*, taking us from one mountain of success to the next upper level. Every peak reached is a success and, as soon as I reach one, I look forward to the next. I strongly believe that we all belong on the peak, straining for the next.

Like many of you, I sometimes fall victim to oppression or enticement, determined to satisfy my inner desires because I did not possess the tools to be in full control of my own soul. But I continue striving as a scholar to possess the vast knowledge of life. Learning is an endless process.

If I enunciate, act, or do something that seems unpleasant to you, I seek refuge in your clemency. I deeply desire to present my passion in a way that all can understand and that offends none.

Let us embrace all our differences and offer leniency for mistakes and accidental misconduct as we strive to leave behind a legacy for upcoming generations.

We live in a world of miracles, surrounded by miracles. We cannot see them, but surely feel and sense them. These miracles fill the universe with infinite energy that keep us alive and healthy. We need to correlate our bodies and souls to align with the Divine Power carrying the Infinite Intelligence beyond our limits.

I finally confess that I am dedicated to living in my own invisible world, *Riding the Endless Cruise of Life (RECL)*, seeking to take every individual step and ride out my journey in sharing the marvels of all PEMS—physical, emotional, mental, and spiritual—aspects of life.

ACKNOWLEDGMENTS

Who are you? What is your value as a human being?

You are a piece of a miracle creature.
Your being glows, this interlinking of subconscious and conscious vitalities.
You are a celestial soul, an immortal spirit.
The whole universe, our galaxy, our beautiful planet Earth,
is surrounded by an Infinite Intelligence that interconnects
your subconscious and conscious potency.
Our world is truly a beautiful paradise,
created and maintained by those who left formidable legacies.
By those who have played a boundless role by climbing the endless mountains of life.

My beloved family and friends have served with me on the front line with motivation and unforgettable support.

Thank you Greta Slabach for all the effort that went into the preliminary editing part of this book.

Thank you Gloria Repp for your full support in making this book come to life.

My highest accolades to the following organizations: the Indian Board of Alternative Medicines (IBAM); the American Holistic Health Association (AHHA); the Academy of Integrative Health & Medicine (AIHM) of the United States; the American Academy for the Advancement in Science (AAAS); Naturopathy 2017 of Australia; Addiction Research & Therapy 2018 of San Diego, CA; the Oman American Business Center –Oman AmCham (OABC); the Sandhya Maarga Holistic Living Academy of Malaysia; the World Yoga Foundation of India; the Philippines College for the Advancement in Medicines (PCAM); Islamic Psychology (IP), Germany; the Pragyan

Pyramid Meditation & Healing Center, India; Virginia Tech Corporate Research Center (VTCRC), Virginia; Edward Via College of Osteopathic Medicine (VCOM), Virginia; Virginia Tech Foundation (VTF), Virginia; VT Outreach International, Virginia; NRV Economic Development; Redeemer Presbyterian Church, Virginia; University of Frères Mentouri Constantine, Algeria.

Thank you for all those organizations that have endowed us with innumerable awards and academic support that gave us the opportunity to present our research and findings.

Thank you to Edward Via College of Osteopathic Medicine (VCOM) for keeping your promises to conduct the first clinical research study on the effectiveness of Haqua Revitalize® Therapy (HART) in human subjects, despite many challenges that have been impeding this clinical study to take place; your continuous promises were always to overcome these challenges and start this clinical study at earliest possible.

What an accomplishment and honor to work on the final stages of this project with the Virginia Tech Corporate Research Center (VTCRC). Thank you for all your efforts.

Thank you to all those who offered their support and belief in Haqua Revitalize® Therapy, since the first day I discovered the effect of hot water at that specific temperature and methodology that was the secret key to magnificent achievements, where personally, I was finally proclaimed by the Royal Oman Police Hospital Medical Committee, being fully asymptomatic from all the chronic ailments that were about to destroy my whole life, by only drinking eight glasses of hot water daily without any medications.

"The doctor of the future will give no medicine but will interest his patients in the care of the human frame, in diet and in the cause and prevention of disease."
-Thomas A. Edison

"Osteopathic medicine focuses on the whole person, the relationship of the body's nerves, muscles, bones and organs, and the body's innate ability to heal itself."
-American Osteopathic Association

"An individual is a whole made up of interdependent parts, which are the physical, mental, emotional, and spiritual. When one part is not working at its best, it impacts all of the other parts of that person."
-American Holistic Health Association

"A living cell requires energy not only for all its functions, but also for the maintenance of its structure... bring out the fact that our body really only knows one fuel, hydrogen. Without energy, life would be extinguished instantaneously, and the cellular fabric would collapse."
-Albert Szent-Györgyi (1937 Nobel Prize Speech.)

"The existing medical establishment is responsible for killing and permanently injuring millions of Americans."
-Dr. Mercola, Osteopathic Physician

What is the reason behind the absence of the symmetrical trend between scientific and technological development and comprehensive human health?

Where is the harmony between scientific and technological development with human health?

Why, on the one hand, are we seeing a revolution of science and technology like never before—

while, when looking at the overall disease and human health statistics in general, we see the trend towards the opposite!

Is it not because of a human being transformed into a laboratory that fills his body with all kinds of toxic chemicals and waste?

Is it not now, before it is too late, to start taking full care of our health and well-being, especially after it was discovered what this easy, cheap and affordable material has carried, as mentioned by MBC in 2012?

Is this aforementioned natural substance not the primary fuel for the body in order to carry its potential toward self-healing, self-protection, and self-maintenance?

This natural substance you know personally. The decision is in your hands.

The modern world is witnessing unprecedented developments in all scientific, cultural, and social fields. On the other hand, the field of human health seems to be losing momentum. There are more medicines and procedures available than ever before, but there are also more ailments and diseases. The number of people turning to ancient traditions and cultures to find a cure is increasing. Natural treatments are growing in popularity at an astounding rate.

Some are rediscovered. Some need further scientific research. And some exist in plain sight.

Haqua, "Hot Water," is one of these. This divine fluid holds vast secrets as the source of the creation and development of every human being. Its potential has altered the direction of the human *PEMS*— physical, emotional, mental, and spiritual—aspects of health.

All matter is made up of atoms: the entire universe, our earth planet, and the human body. The formation of a human body begins with a single cell. At the point of birth, one cell has become seventy trillion. A single cell is made up of one hundred trillion atoms and an atom is made up of electrons, protons, and neutrons. The *PEMS*—physical, emotional, mental, and emotional—aspects of health in every individual relies on the health of these cells. Fifty to seventy billion cells in an adult die every day and replacement cells must be produced. The cell cycle is a marvel of life.

Depletion of the *Four Essential Elements of Life (FEELs)*—water, oxygen, hydrogen, and energy— is responsible for all abnormal functions in the human body. Therefore, much research has been conducted on water, oxygen, hydrogen, and energy therapies. Because each cell of the human body relies on these unique elements, *Haqua Revitalize® Therapy (HART)* combines all four of them. In their individual format, the above therapies limit the health benefits available.

The *Four Essential Elements of Life (FEELs)* are not available in their complete form from any other source than *Haqua Revitalize® Therapy (HART)*.

Other names of *Haqua Revitalize® Therapy (HART)*:

- Hot Aqua Therapy (HAT),
- Hydro-Thermal Therapy (HTT),
- Aqua Calidum Therapy (ACT),
- Aqua Thermal Therapy (ATT),
- May Sakhin Therapy (MST),
- Maji Moto Therapy (MMT),
- Hot Water Therapy (HWT).

This innovative approach to holistic health possesses the ability to transform natural health and wellbeing, while revitalizing the human's *PEMS*—physical, emotional, mental, and spiritual—aspects.

According to the American Holistic Health Association, an individual is made up of interdependent parts, the *PEMS* aspects of life. When one part is dysfunctional, the whole person is impacted.

Andrew Taylor Still, MD, DO—founder of osteopathy and osteopathic medicine—laid especial emphasis on the self-regulation, self-tenets healing, and health maintenance capabilities of the human body.

The *Four Essential Elements of Life (FEELs)* generate health through the use of the *BICADU*—Believe, Implement, Continue, Appreciate, Discipline, understand—principles of *Haqua Revitalize® Therapy (HART)*.

These are the missing puzzle pieces in healthcare, with the potential to carry out two basic, but essential, functions: naturally destroying pathogenic bacteria, toxins, and the poisonous products of organisms, and melting fat in the body by enhancing the enzymes that break up the deposits into reusable resources—amino acids from proteins, fatty acids from fats, glucose from carbohydrates. Both fatty acids and glucose are needed by the cells as sources of energy, and amino acids are necessary for cell energy and building muscle and body tissues.

The recommended temperature of Haqua 'hot water' used in all the therapeutic modalities differs depending on the age of the subject to assure appropriate thermogenesis and secure proper vein vasodilation.

Haqua Revitalize® Therapy (HART) is a natural, toxin-free dietary supplement for people of all ages and races with enormous benefits that has the potential to revitalize human biological and genetic structures. The therapeutic benefits resulting from this therapy are extensive.

As shown in this chart, we have observed the following results for technological growth versus health decline:

The human body is created with systems to address and destroy harmful substances, but the high level of toxic matter has caused these systems to break down.

With the proper supply of the *Four Essential Elements of Life (FEELs)*, all of which are offered through *Haqua Revitalize® Therapy (HART)*, humanity will once more find full health in every aspect of life.

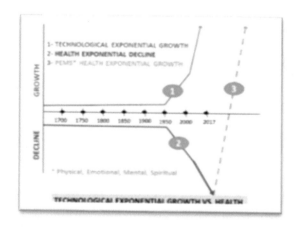

The research conducted on the elements offered through this therapy will finally solve the multiple controversies over nutrition, dieting, exercise, detoxing, sunbathing, etc.

As humanity becomes more aware of their health requirements and how to naturally supply them, there will be less of a need for conventional medications and procedures. Each person will be able to address their own personal needs and then live life fully without continually relying on surgeries and drugs.

The discovery of Haqua Revitalize® Therapy (HART) will regenerate and reshape civilization. Health is the most prominent wealth any person could have the privilege to achieve, and the time to start is now.

Faris AlHajri- Ph.D. (A.M.)

PREFACE

My dearly beloved mother—may her soul rest in peace—lived her entire life with numerous health complications. From the time I was two years old, she had suffered from the same disease for more than thirty years and had undergone ten surgical operations in her stomach—seven in Africa, and three in the United Kingdom.

In my family, I am second to youngest of eight children. Because my mother's health made it impossible for her to care for us, my siblings and I were split between two paternal uncles who lived in different towns in the eastern part of Congo. My parents lived in a nearby country. As a result, I always considered my auntie and uncle "Mom" and "Dad."

One day, while playing in the home garden, I was informed that my true parents had arrived for a short holiday from the country in which they were living; I was just six years old at that time. This sudden news caused conflicting emotions for me. I ran in to see them, shocked and confused, wondering how I could have two mothers and two fathers.

Such meetings were sporadic, due to the health conditions of my mother. Many years passed between visits and those visits lasted only a short amount of time.

During one of these visits, as I was running down the long corridor of my uncle's house to see my parents, I crashed with my elder sister at the corridor corner. She was carrying a tea pot full of boiled milk tea. The scalding liquid spilled over both of us, resulting in first-degree burns. Laid out on chairs, our shirts were removed, peeling off a layer of skin at the same time. A mixture of salt and oil was then applied. Both of us were in terrible pain and I didn't get a chance to hug my parents.

This unpleasant incident and the resulting scars haunted me for the rest of my youth, evolving into a chronic inferiority complex. I always preferred to be alone and deeply admired and appreciated nature. Frequently outdoors, I enjoyed the rain and sitting in elevated places, searching for the uncertain.

Where I lived, night brought an extraordinary blanket of stars spread on a velvet canvas. I loved to watch the stars and dream. My deepest aspiration was to make my dreams and wishes come true when I grow older: finding a permanent cure for my mother with no side effects, and then living with my real parents.

Unfortunately, my mother passed away before I was able to find a cure for her, but I am grateful that we all got to be near her when her last hours came.

As a workaholic, I immersed myself in very long hours of non-stop work, constantly searching for the uncertain, and thus I suffered for many years with various chronic diseases: allergic rhinitis, asthma, migraines, and lumbago. Living with these diseases for so many years, and the frequent use of medications, caused my health to go from bad to worse. This resulted in a health phobia, as I obsessed over what had happened to my mother. What if the same scenario happened to me? There was no hope of permanently curing any of my diseases, nor even of real improvement. The doctors kept repeating that my diseases were already chronic, incurable, and that I would have to live with them my entire life.

Nonetheless, I intensified my efforts through personal experimentation and exploration. I tried various forms of alternative medicine, particularly Ayurveda, but nothing was helping.

Finally, two interconnected incidents occurred that completely changed my life forever. The first was a dream sometime in April 2007. I awakened from this powerful and unimaginable vision early in the morning and realized that it was not just a dream, but a powerful subconscious vitality penetrating my brain. After experiencing this powerful brainstorm, I promptly woke my wife Gloria and started talking as fast as I could. The only assurance that I could give her of my coming revelation was *"just wait and see."*

The second event came four months after the first incident. My discovery of *Haqua Revitalize® Therapy*, publicly known as Hot Water Therapy, using experimentation of cold and boiled water on leftover oils on our dishes, was caused by that same mysterious brainstorm that came before. That was the beginning of an evolution of health that will revitalize the world with the promise of a natural, toxin-free substance that exists anywhere humans live. This is the secret of complete human health.

As a quantity surveyor (a construction industry professional responsible for managing all aspects of the contractual and financial side of construction projects) with experience in managing government projects for twenty years, I neither had any knowledge about holistic health and wellness in particular, nor about health in general. The only thing I had was phobia, fear, and reiterated worries of getting sick. It all started with repetitively reading numerous articles about health, food, and environment. That is where I first came across information about the adverse effects of carbohydrates, cold water, etc. I then decided to avoid eating rice and drinking cold water, and did so for many years. But that was not enough to protect me from accounting these various chronic diseases.

After the story of my complete cure from these chronic ailments I encountered, most especially, the complete medical check-up that covered vital signs: blood pressure, heart rate, respiratory rate; the visual exam which covered head, eyes, chest, abdomen, nervous system functions; physical exams from eyes, ears and nose; and full laboratory tests. All the test results were astonishing, and the issue was raised to the Medical Committee of the Royal Oman Police Hospital, where my wife used to work as a registered nurse: and I was granted a certificate for having been cured from all my chronic ailments and I was found asymptomatic.

The following step was to fulfill my dream to heal the world, so I started sharing my story to the public, and I started receiving testimonials from those who were following my guidelines.

The only choice left to me, as media started inviting me to share my story after I wrote my first book, was to change professions. I had to step out of my professional work of Quantity Surveying and my latest position as Technical Expert in the office of Undersecretary of Ministry of Housing, even though my position in the government was my highest ever achieved. When I tendered my resignation, the Minister of Housing refused it. I had to insist, and to convince him, I told him the world needs me as well; for what I recently discovered, there would be a very long journey I needed to go through to achieve my childhood passion, dream and ambition. Later, I found I first needed to study holistic health and wellness, and engage with like-minded professionals through international conferences as a speaker in my topic. Fortunately, my resignation was automatically turned to early pension based upon my years of serving my job: a contingency that would help me support my family in times of any financial crisis that may occur due to this act.

The biggest challenge was whenever I was invited to give a live television interview, or conduct a lecture in secondary school, followed by universities like the University of the Philippines, and Oman's Sultan Qaboos University. I had to carefully prepare the topic of my presentation. How could I do that, when I was just a quantity surveyor? I never had any academic, or even scientific training in holistic health, nor alternative medicine. I was even confused about which area of science Hot Water Therapy, which I later dubbed *Haqua Revitalize® Therapy*, would fit! The only knowledge I had was from the articles I'd been reading for several years about cold water side effects, the Japanese and American water therapies, and a few about nutrition, such as the controversy about the adverse health effects of carbohydrates, fizzy drinks, etc. It was one of the biggest challenges I ever faced, the highest and toughest mountain among which I coined the "endless mountains of life." I was fully determined to climb it, whatever the cost and challenges I would face. My story is too long; to keep short, I kept a credit to write my autobiography in a complete separate book, to be launched in the near future.

To pursue my vision of writing my books, after I successfully wrote two books in two languages at the same time,

I was working hard to finalize my two upcoming new books: *Haqua Revitalize® Therapy – The Lost Treasure* and *The Power of You – Amplify Your Subconscious Vitality* when I became deeply concerned with the recent Coronavirus (COVID-19) outbreak.

This reminded me of two important incidents the universe was trying to show me, to realize this was something that needs intensive attention; these two incidents happened as follows:

- ❖ The first incident reminded me what happened during my family trip to Asia in summer of 2009, when suddenly a novel influenza A (H1N1) virus emerged, which became a flu pandemic or swine flu. As we were on our trip to a cruise, I was attacked with a terrible cold, cough, and severe headache; all those were the signs of the swine flu infection. On our return from the cruise to our hotel, it became so serious that I decided not to report to the authorities, thinking I would be put under quarantine and ruin all our travel plans. I asked my sister and her two daughters, who were with us in our trip, sleep in a room along with my wife. I completely isolated myself for twenty-four hours, and all throughout the night, I kept drinking plenty of hot water—a half-liter (17 oz.) every half hour—along with doing the steam and compress methods. I needed the toilet every 10-20 minutes, and sometimes I was vomiting, and kept passing loose bowel movements, with terrible abdominal pain involved. However, by the time twenty-four hours passed, though I did not sleep overnight, I was overwhelmed to have fully recovered. For this reason, I devoted to share the methodologies I used when I was infected with such an exclusive ailment that carried all the symptoms of the Swine Flu (H1N1), which may help in dealing with the outbreak of Coronavirus (COVID-19). Thus, I would strongly recommend you abide with the rules and regulations of the health authorities and your physician while using our *Haqua Revitalize® Therapy (HART)* as recommended here in this book. We strongly recommend you read our disclaimer as mentioned in the forefront pages of this book.

❖ The other incident was the recent clinical research study that was conducted by a group of students from the University of Frères Mentouri Constantine on the effect of hot water on inflammation induced by hypercholesterolemia in rats (Chapter 2: Clinical Study – Université les Frères Mentouri, Constantine).

The potential spread of the Coronavirus (COVID-19) started causing intense, widespread impacts to the global economy as more and more people became infected with the virus.

Thus, my wife Gloria wisely convinced me to write an article or post a video on the effect of Haqua Revitalize® in dealing with COVID-19. She got very active trying to contact various media outlets in the US—the *Washington Post*, CNN, the *New York Times*, and even the Office of the President of the United States and the Oman Embassy in Washington D.C.—pleading to them and referring them to more than five hundred sources of anecdotal evidence we collected from beneficiaries; our entire family living in full healthy condition since the discovery of hot water therapy; and moreover, the recent clinical research study conducted in Algeria as mentioned. Here, she convinced me to fully focus on publishing this book rather than just meeting the media, and later trying to reach the media after issuing the book on the effect of hot water therapy on COVID-19. This book took me less than a week to write, where I compiled some crucial information from my book *The Lost Treasure* that I was finalizing to readying to launch.

HAQUAPATHY

What is the concept of "Haquapathy"?

The name *"Haquapathy"* is the implementation of the entire *Haqua Revitalize® Therapy*, covering all the internal and external therapeutic modalities.

Haquate *means to make the body absorb the elements found in hot water, coined as the Four Essential Elements of Life (FEELs)*. Haqua *derives from two words: "hot" and "aqua," from the Latin word for water.* Haqua Revitalize® *is the reinstatement of the human body* to its initial state of creation in the precise form of complete PEMS (Physical, Emotional, Mental, and Spiritual) aspects of health, through the implementation of Haqua Revitalize® Therapeutic Modalities (HRTM). The word "-pathy" comes from Latin, mean therapy.

Haquapathy is one of the basic methods of treatment in the system of natural medicine, which is also called Hot Aqua Therapy, Hot Water Therapy, Hydrothermal Therapy, Aqua Calidum Therapy, Maysakhin Therapy, and Majimoto Therapy, instigated by the author, originator and founder of this therapy since he discovered its significant health benefits to the human body in August 2007, until the present moment. Since then, he asserted it as a new part of alternative medicine (particularly naturopathy), that involves the use of Haqua Revitalize® Therapy.

Haquapathic Medicine is a newly introduced form of primary health care profession, emphasizing prevention, treatment, and optimal health through the use of Haqua Revitalize® Therapy toward individuals' inherent self-healing, self-protection and self-maintenance process.

"Life is a School that has an Endless Process of Learning;

Every Day, there is something to Learn, and learn, and Learn."

Faris AlHajri-Ph.D. (A.M.)

Founder of Haquapathic Medicine

Chapter 1

CORONAVIRUS DISEASE 2019 (COVID-19)

Section 1: About COVID-19 outbreak

The coronavirus disease 2019 (COVID-19), which used to be called the novel coronavirus (2019-nCoV), is a new type of coronavirus which causes respiratory illness in people. It was first identified in Wuhan, China. COVID-19 can spread from person to person, which usually happens through respiratory droplets—when someone with the virus coughs or sneezes, and you breathe it in. The symptoms include fever, cough, and shortness of breath.

❖ Many of the people who have a COVID-19 infection have pneumonia in both lungs.

❖ There is a test for COVID-19. There is no vaccine or specific treatment for COVID-19. Medical care can help to relieve the symptoms.

There are several different types of human coronaviruses, including the Middle East respiratory syndrome (MERS) and severe acute respiratory syndrome (SARS) coronaviruses. There are no specific treatments for coronavirus infections. Most people will get better on their own.[1]

As of 27 February 2020, there have been 2,810 confirmed deaths and more than 82,500 confirmed cases in the coronavirus pneumonia outbreak.[2,3,4]

Because this is a new virus, there are still things we do not know, such as how severe the illness can be, how well it is transmitted between people, and other features of the virus. CDC believes that symptoms of COVID-19 may appear two to 14 days after exposure.[5]

The new coronavirus attacks the lungs, and in about 20% of patients, infections can become more serious. As the virus enters lung cells, it starts to replicate, destroying the cells, explains Dr. Yoko Furuya, an infectious disease specialist at Columbia University Irving Medical Center. Furuya says that this immune system response to the invader can also destroy lung tissue and cause inflammation. The end result can be pneumonia—the air sacs in the lungs become inflamed and filled with fluid, making it harder to breathe. Dr. Carlos del Rio, a professor of medicine and global health at Emory University says that these symptoms can also make it harder for the lungs to get oxygen to your blood, potentially triggering a cascade of problems. *"The lack of oxygen leads to more inflammation, more problems in the body. Organs need oxygen to function, right? So when you don't have oxygen there, then your liver dies and your kidney dies,"* he says.

That's what seems to be happening in the most severe cases. About three to five percent of patients end up in intensive care, according to WHO, and many hospitalized patients require supplemental oxygen.

Many of the more serious cases have been in people who are middle-aged and elderly — Furuya notes that our immune systems weaken as we age. She says it could be even worse for long-term smokers, since their airways and lungs are more vulnerable. People with other underlying medical conditions, such as heart disease, diabetes or chronic lung disease, have also proven most vulnerable. Furuya says those kinds of conditions can make it harder for the body to recover from infections.[6]

During infection of the coronavirus COVID-19, high levels of inflammatory cytokines have been reported.[7] Cytokines are small secreted proteins released by cells which affect the interactions and communications between cells. There are both pro-inflammatory cytokines and anti-inflammatory cytokines. Cytokines act in concert with specific cytokine inhibitors and soluble cytokine receptors to regulate the human immune response.[8]

When liver cells are inflamed or damaged, they can leak higher than normal amounts of enzymes into the bloodstream. One recent report published in the *Lancet Journals* found signs of liver damage in a person with COVID-19. Doctors says it's not clear, though, if the virus or the medication being used to treat the person caused the damage. With any infection, the body's immune system responds by attacking the foreign virus or bacteria. While this immune response can rid the body of the infection, it can also sometimes cause collateral damage in the body. This can come in the form of an intense inflammatory response, sometimes called a "cytokine storm." The immune cells produce cytokines to fight infection, but if too many are released, it can cause problems in the body.[9]

How may Haqua Revitalize Therapy® help treating Coronavirus (COVID-19)?

Haquate means to make the body absorb water, oxygen, hydrogen and energy (WOHE). These elements have been found to be the body's essential fuels. We coined them *the Four Essential Elements of Life (FEELs). Haquate* derives from *Haqua. Haqua Revitalize*® is the reinstatement of the human body to its initial state of creation in the precise form of complete physical, emotional, mental, and spiritual (PEMS) aspects of health. The three tenets of Osteopathic Medicine, which express its underlying philosophy, are: the body is capable of self-regulation, self-healing, and health maintenance.[10] The human body's immune system would gradually start crumpling the moment it is depleted from one or more of its essential fuels, the *FEELs*. A 2017 thesis submitted by students for the degree of Master of Immuno-oncology from the University of Frères Mentouri Constantine in Algeria, on the effects of hot water on inflammation induced by hypercholesterolemia in rats, by conducting a peer review of our recommended consumption of hot water[11] concluded as follows:

❖ The recommended consumption of hot water play a role on the body weight, and it has an anti-inflammatory effect for long or short term. So the use of hot water seems to have an interest in prevention of atherosclerosis and inflammatory bowel disease (IBD).

❖ The present experimental finding showed that hot water therapy process has a positive effect on the inflammation and a decrease in lipids status.

❖ We considered that the hot water is a natural hydrotherapy during the short or long term, dependent on type of disease. [12]

Section 2: Exceptional Haqua Gulping (TMHG) for COVID-19

1st Day (In Full Isolation)

➤ Drink a glass/mug/tumbler of 500 ml/17 oz up to one liter/34 oz of Hot Water (Haqua) at 1-2 hours intervals – highly advised to reach five liters (169 oz) at 50°C/122° F within the first 24 hours.

➤ Full Hot Water Fasting – Refrain completely from eating or drinking anything besides hot water as mentioned above

➤ Apply both Haqua Compress Method (HCM) and Haqua Steam Method (HSM) whenever possible, as recommended (▶See Sections 3 and 4)

➤ Abide your physician's instructions (medical doctor), strictly follow his/her advice

2nd and 3rd Days (In Full Isolation)

➤ Drink a glass/mug/tumbler of 500 ml/17 oz up to one liter/34 oz of Hot Water (Haqua) at two-hour intervals – highly advised between 3-4 liters/101-135 oz at 50° C/122° F.

➤ Full Liquid Diet – No solid foods at all, and only consume liquids such as hot soups, besides hot water as mentioned above

➤ Apply both Haqua Compress Method (HCM) and Haqua Steam Method (HSM) whenever possible, as recommended (▶See Sections 3 and 4).

➤ Abide by your physician's instructions (medical doctor): strictly follow his/her advice.

4th Day through 2 weeks, or until recovery (In Full Isolation)

➤ Drink a glass/mug/tumbler of 500 ml/17 oz up to one liter/34 oz of Hot Water (Haqua) at two hour intervals – highly advised between 3-4 liters/101-135 oz at 50° C/122° F.

➤ Half Liquid Diet – Limit solid foods and consume liquids, such as hot soups, besides hot water as mentioned above on the second day.

- ➢ Apply both Haqua Compress Method (HCM) and Haqua Steam Method (HSM) whenever possible, as recommended (▶See Sections 3 and 4).

- ➢ Abide by your physician's instructions (medical doctor): strictly follow his/her advice.

After 2 weeks (until fully recovered)

- ➢ Follow the Haqua Common Gulping Method (HCGM)-For Adults as recommended (▶See Section 5).

- ➢ Full Liquid Diet – No solid foods and only consume liquids, such as hot soups, besides hot water as mentioned above

- ➢ Apply both Haqua Compress Method (HCM) and Haqua Steam Method (HSM) whenever possible, as recommended (▶See Sections 3 and 4).

- ➢ Abide by your physician's instructions (medical doctor): strictly follow his/her advice.

Section 3: Haqua Compress Method (HCM)

Option I (recommended)

- ➢ Boil water in a wireless water boiler and place it in a safe area near your shower.

- ➢ Take a hot shower and thoroughly clean your body.

- ➢ After showering, pour hot water from the shower tap into a small container or basin with similar size of the water boiler filling only ¾ of the container.

- ➢ Add boiled water from the water boiler to the container or basin.

- ➢ Immerse a small towel (approximately 30cmx30cm/1ftx1ft in size) halfway or fully in the basin filled with Haqua (hot water). Maintain a temperature of around 70°C-80°C/160°F-180°F in the basin.

- ➢ Test the temperature of the wet towel with your hand. Make sure that it is not too hot.

➢ Gently rub and massage all parts of your body, following the Therapeutic Steps below. Each part should be done once or twice. After each step, re-wet your towel. This will maintain a steady heat throughout the process.

➢ Keep refilling the container or basin every time there is no more hot water same as earlier explained.

➢ The overall process should take around four minutes.

➢ It is recommended to use this therapy once daily, four to five days per week.

➢ Two towels will be needed.

Therapeutic Steps: Towel 1

➢ Face.

➢ Neck.

➢ Right shoulder, covering the front and back parts of your shoulder.

➢ Left shoulder, covering the front and back parts of your shoulder.

➢ Right hand up to the fingers.

➢ Left hand up to the fingers.

➢ Chest down to the stomach.

➢ Right leg down to the ankle.

➢ Left leg down to the ankle.

➢ Right foot, covering the tops and bottoms of the foot and toes.

➢ Left foot, covering the tops and bottoms of the foot and toes.

Therapeutic Steps: Towel 2

> ➤ Apply to the genital part of your body.

The Haqua Compress Method is recommended to be performed by a professional Holistic Health Therapist or Massage Therapist in this field to prevent injury.

Option II

> ➤ Take a hot shower and thoroughly clean your body.

> ➤ Using a small towel (approximately 30cmx30cm/1ftx1ft in size), increase the temperature of the water. As the hot water continues to run, gently rub your body, following the steps mentioned hereinbefore.

Section 4: Haqua Steam Method (HSM)

Therapeutic Methods for personal or home use

> ➤ Fill one third of an electric water boiler with clean tap water and cover as much of the body as possible with a blanket or towel.

> ➤ Boil the water and keep the cover of the electric boiler opened.

> ➤ Keep the steam at a temperature that does not burn your face.

> ➤ Inhale the steam with your mouth and release it through the nose. Then inhale with your nose and release through your mouth.

> ➤ Inhale from one side of your nose and release the steam through the other side of your nose, and vice versa.

> ➤ Use this method for around 4 minutes.

> ➤ The Haqua Steam Method is recommended to be performed by a professional Holistic Health Therapist or Massage Therapist in this field to prevent injury.

Section 5: Haqua Common Gulping Method (HCGM)-For Adults

Otherwise known as Therapeutic Methods of Haqua Gulping (TMHG).

TMHG, publicly known as the Therapeutic Methods of Drinking Hot Water (TMDHW). The Haqua Common Gulping Method (HCGM), as recommended for adults with glass size 500 ml/17 oz, should be as follows:

1. One glass upon waking and on a 'clean' mouth* – at a standing position.

2. One glass between 7:00-10:00 a.m.

3. One glass 15-30 minutes before lunch. **

4. One glass between 2:00-4:00 p.m.

5. One glass in the evening, 15-30 minutes before dinner. **

6. One glass an hour before sleep. **

Notes:

Haqua should be taken before brushing teeth, mouthwash, or eating anything.

** Should be given high consideration. *Haqua* will detoxify the body, removing toxins which are in the form of gases (Carbon Dioxide-CO_2, Hydrogen Sulfide-H_2S, Nitrogen-N, and Methane-CH_4).

➤ The Therapeutic Methods of Haqua Gulping (TMHG) as revealed here, is quite similar to that mentioned in Chapter 2: Clinical Study: University of Frères Mentouri Constantine: Option 1 – Drinking Method for glass size 500 ml. In this session, it has been simplified to make it much easier to remember and apply.

➤ The daily recommended consumption of Haqua (Hot Water) is a minimum of three liters (101 oz) and maximum of four liters (135 oz).

➢ The water volume consumed should not exceed 500 ml (17 oz) at one time, and a maximum of one liter in the span of an hour.

➢ The recommended temperature of Haqua is fixed at around 50ºC (122ºF), a little bit less than the temperature of hot tea or hot coffee.

➢ There are several other gulping methods that suit the daily activity for individuals, and other gulping methods and the water temperature in accordance to age, from toddlers, babies, children, and adolescents as well.

➢ The regular method for testing the temperature of Haqua is recommended by being able to fill up your mouth at one gulp without burning.

➢ It is important that the maximum temperature of the Haqua is maintained at 50ºC (122ºF) so that the availability of hydrogen, oxygen, and energy is high.

➢ A whole tumbler of size of 500 ml (17 oz) is highly recommended every 2-3 hours.

➢ Boiled water can be mixed with warm or cold water to reach the desired temperature as recommended.

➢ Water can be heated up by any method available to you: water heater, water dispenser, microwave, wood stove, electric boiler, gas for heating, etc.

➢ Do not exceed more than a 3-hour interval without drinking, except in urgent and exceptional cases.

➢ Do not gulp more than one liter (34 oz) Haqua within one hour.

➢ It is strongly recommended not to mix your *Haqua* (hot water) with any additives. Any change of water's temperature, or addition of additives, immediately alters its molecular state, and it can even become toxic.

➢ Because the body will rid itself of toxins, there may be a few unpleasant side effects. This, however, is a natural result and a healthy response to Haqua's cleansing work. The detoxification process includes excreting metabolic wastes, accumulated toxins, harmful bacteria and excess fat deposits (lipids).

➢ There may be some irregular stomach discharge, frequent urination and sweating. This symptom usually lasts for a week or two (more or less) before the body is revitalized and returns to its normal condition.

➢ Some vomiting is possible and may continue one or two times while the body detoxes.

References (Chapter 1)

1. Coronavirus Infections. MedlinePlus. U.S. National Library of Medicine. https://medlineplus.gov/coronavirusinfections.html - accessed February 28, 2020.

2. "Operations Dashboard for ArcGIS". gisanddata.maps.arcgis.com. The Center for Systems Science and Engineering (CSSE) is a research collective housed within the Department of Civil and Systems Engineering (CaSE) at Johns Hopkins University (JHU). 28 January 2020. Archived from the original on 28 January 2020. Retrieved 3 February 2020.

3. "Coronavirus Toll Update: Cases & Deaths by Country of Wuhan, China Virus - Worldometer". www.worldometers.info. Archived from the original on 2 February 2020. Retrieved 2 February 2020.

4. Coronavirus. Wikipedia the free encyclopedia. https://en.wikipedia.org/wiki/Coronavirus - accessed February 28, 2020.

5. About Coronavirus Disease 2019 (COVID-19). Minnesota Department of Health. https://www.health.state.mn.us/diseases/coronavirus/basics.html - accessed February 28, 2020.

6. How COVID-19 Kills: The New Coronavirus Disease Can Take A Deadly Turn. NPR Radio. Maria Godoy. February 14, 2020. Weekend Edition Sunday. https://www.npr.org/sections/goatsandsoda/2020/02/14/805289669/how-covid-19-kills-the-new-coronavirus-disease-can-take-a-deadly-turn - accessed February 28, 2020.

7. Fighting Against Coronavirus. Research Products for COVID-19 (SARS-CoV-2). RayBiotech. https://www.raybiotech.com/coronavirus-research-products-sars-cov-2-covid-19/- accessed February 28, 2020.

8. Zhang JM, An J. Cytokines, inflammation, and pain. Int Anesthesiol Clin. 2007 Spring;45(2):27-37. doi: 10.1097/AIA.0b013e318034194e. PMID: 17426506; PMCID: PMC2785020.- https://www.ncbi.nlm.nih.gov/pmc/articles/PMC2785020/ - accessed March 01, 2020

9. Here's What Happens to the Body After Contracting the Coronavirus. Shawn Radcliffe. February 20, 2020. https://www.healthline.com/health-news/heres-what-happens-to-the-body-after-contracting-the-coronavirus - accessed February 28, 2020.

10. Tenets of Osteopathic Medicine. American osteopathic Association. https://osteopathic.org/about/leadership/aoa-governance-documents/tenets-of-osteopathic-medicine/ - accessed February 28, 2020.

11. AlHajri Faris. (2010). The miracle & wonders of treatment from hot water: hot water miracles. 1-108. https://www.farisalhajri.com

12. The effects of hot water on inflammation induced by hypercholesterolemia in rats. University of Frères Mentouri Constantine. Ministry of Higher Education and Scientific Research. Guennoub S, Redouane R, Dr Messoudi s, Pr Zerizer S, Dr Aribi B. http://fac.umc.edu.dz/snv/faculte/biblio/mmf/2017/The%20Effect%20of%20hot%20water%20on%20inflammation%20induced%20by%20hypercholesterolemia%20in%20rats.pdf - accessed February 28, 2020.

Chapter 2

CLINICAL STUDY: UNIVERSITY OF FRÈRES MENTOURI CONSTANTINE

This clinical research study was conducted by a group of students at the University of Frères Mentouri Constantine in Algeria, for their Master's degree thesis under the supervision of Professor Zerizer Sakina.[12]

Further clarifications of this thesis are provided at the end of this chapter. Only parts of the thesis were provided here. For the entire thesis, refer to the link provided above at the end of Chapter 1.

The Effect of Hot Water on Inflammation Induced by Hypercholesterolemia in Rats

Abbreviations

CHD	**: Coronary Heart Disease**	**CRP**	**: C-Reactive Protein**
CVD	: Cardiovascular Disease	**CD**	: Crohn's Disease
FA	: Fatty Acid	**FH**	: Familial Hypercholesterolemia
GI	: Gastrointestinal Tract	**HDL**	: High Density Lipoprotein

HMG-CoA	: Hydroxyl-Methylglutaryl -Coenzyme A	**IDL**	: Intermediate Density Lipoprotein
IBD	: Inflammatory Bowel Disease	**LDL**	: Low Density Lipoprotein
MUFA	: Monounsaturated Fatty Acid	**Ox-LDL**	: Oxidized LDL
PUFA	: Polyunsaturated Fatty Acid	**ROS**	: Reactive Oxygen Species
SFA	: Saturated Fatty Acid	**SMCs**	: Smooth Muscle Cells
TFA	: Trans Fatty Acid	**T- CH**	: Total Cholesterol
TG	: Triglyceride	**UC**	: Ulcerative Colitis
VLDL	: Very Low Density Lipoprotein		

Hot Water purifies the toxin, helps melting the fat deposits and destroys harmful bacteria in our body. It is the most important catalyst in losing weight, it can also help the gastrointestinal tract to function even better. It's get rid of fat, reduce obesity, and cured high blood cholesterol, Stroke, Gastroenteritis, Heart Disease **(AlHajri, 2010).**

Objectives

➤ Evaluate the effect of saturated, Trans-fatty acids and hot water on the weight and diet of rats.

➤ Evaluate the effect of hot water on hypercholesterolemia induced by Trans-fats by measuring the levels of T-Ch., HDL-c, LDL-c and TG.

➤ Evaluate the effect of hot water on the inflammation by measuring C-reactive protein induced by hypercholesterolemia.

The Miracle and Wonder of Treatment with Hot Water

Heat is the only element that destroy harmful bacteria, melts the fats and neutralizes the toxins that spread in our bodies from the food preservative today's world. The only means to split H with O by heating water which will there after burn the O from water in a form of odorless and colorless, however, drinking at least (8) glasses of hot water daily, with enough heat affordable for our bodies. We end up inhaling a large quantity of H, which considered as the main body's nutrient element **(AlHajri, 2010)**.

Benefits of Drinking Hot Water

Prevent various diseases, symptoms and allergies. Heal people in pain, with sickness, allergies and diseases even if how critical it is. Get rid of fat. Reduce obesity, heals bronchial asthma, diabetes, hypertension, high cholesterol… etc., Improve brain memory. Possess a good-looking body. To be healthy, we must drink the required quantity of Hot Water in a day. Health is wealth, so we have to keep a healthy body to have a wealthy lifestyle **(AlHajri, 2010)**.

Materials

Animals

The experiment was performed on 20 males young wistar albino rats, (1-2 Months) weighing between (57.1g-126.7g). All animals were born in animal house (university des frères Mentouri Constantine), and they were housed in cages with free access to water and diet every day at room temperature.

Blood samples

After 21 days of experiment, animals were fasted overnight and the blood was obtained from the retro orbital sinus and collected into EDTA tubes.

Methods

Biochemical analysis

Treatment of rats

After acclimatization to the laboratory conditions for 10 days, the twenty rats were divided into four groups and fed for 21 days with control and experimental diets.

All animals in the groups I (C) *"normal water + animal diet"* and IV (HW) *"Hot water + Animal Diet"* were fed with animal diets however the groups II (CH/W) *"Normal water + Animal diet + Trans-fats"* and III (CH/HW) *"Hot water + Animal diet + Trans-fats"* were fed with diet rich in trans-fats, the groups I *"Normal water + Animal Diet"* and II *"Normal water + Animal diet + Trans-fats"* have drink normal water but III *"Hot water + Animal diet + Trans-fats"* and IV *"Hot water + Animal Diet"* have drink hot water (around 50°C) (table 10), the animals were kept in cages, the weight and diet and water consumed by rats were taken throughout the experiment at the same time. After 21days, the animals were fasted overnight, and the blood was collected for biochemical analysis.

Materials and methods

Table 02: Composition of diet taken by rats during 21 days

Animal diet	Trans fats material		
Corn	Chips (6g per day)		
Soy	Vegetable oil (10g)		
Barley	Cheese (6g per day)		
Cellulose	Cake (12g per day)		
Minerals			
Vitamins			

Table 03: Treatment of rats for 21 days

Experimental Group	Treatment	Number Of Animals	Duration Of Experiment	Daily Dose
GI(C)	Normal water + Animal Diet	5	21	175ml/5rats
GII (CH/W)	Normal water + Animal Diet + Trans fats	5	21	175ml + 34g/5rats
GIII(CH/HW)	Hot water + Animal Diet + Trans fats	5	21	175ml + 34g/5rats
GIV(HW)	Hot water + Animal Diet	5	21	175ml/5rats

2.1. b. Lipids Determination

The objective of lipids determination is to detect the hypercholesterolemia. Total cholesterol, HDL-c, LDL-c, and triglyceride were measured using colorimetric automatic procedures (Auto-Analyzer type Roche Integra 400) at laboratory of AL AMINE Constantine.

2.1. c. High Sensitivity C-reactive protein (hs-CRP) determination

The Objective of hs-CRP measurement is to evaluate the possibility of infection or inflammatory disease. The plasma hs-CRP values were measured by [immunoturbidimetric] method on auto-analyzer (laboratory AL Alamine).

2.2. Histological analysis

After blood samples collection, the animals were kept in the laboratory for another extra 5 days of treatment, the G I (C) *"Normal water + Animal Diet"* and G IV (HW) *"Hot water + Animal Diet"* were fed with animal diet and supplemented with bread and they have drink normal water and hot water respectively, however the groups II *"Hot water + Animal diet + Trans-fats"* and III *"Hot water + Animal diet + Trans-fats"* they were fed with diet rich in trans fats and supplemented with animal fats which is source of saturated fatty acids and bread and they have drink normal and hot water respectively (Table04). Then after this period of twenty six days of the experimental work the animals were sacrificed and organs (liver, heart, aorta, spleen and intestine) dissected and weighed immediately in the wet state. After that some of these samples (liver, heart, aorta and sigmoid colon) were rinsed from all adherent adipose tissue in NaCl (0.9%) then the samples were fixed in formal (10%) for histological investigation.

Table 04: Composition of diet taken by rats during 5extra days of treatment.

Animal diet	Trans fats material
Corn	Chips (6g per day)
Soy	Vegetable oil (10g)
Barley	Cheese (6g per day)
Cellulose	Fats (6g per day)

Minerals	Cake (12g per day)
Vitamins	
Bread	

Results and Discussion

Results

Animal investigations

Diet variation

Control group I (group C)

The diet taken from the group I (C) *"Normal water + Animal Diet"* during the first, second and third week was

(46.71g±1.82), (59.03g±6.56) and (42.63g±9.51) respectively. There is a difference very highly significantly in diet consumption between weeks p= 0.002.

The Tukey's test indicated that the diet consumed by rats in the second week is increased significantly when it is compared to the first week p=0.023. However the diet consumed by rats in the third week is decrease highly significantly when it is compared to the second week p=0.002 (Table05 annex).

Cholesterol/water group II (CH/W) *"Normal water + Animal diet + Trans-fats"*

In the group II (CH/W), the consumption of diet during the first until the third week was (47.16g±5.39), (41.91g±2.19) and (43.32g±22.14) respectively. There is a difference in diet consumption between weeks p=0.806.

The Tukey's test indicated that the diet consumed by rats in the third week is decreased not significantly when compared to the first week p=0.05 (Table06 annex).

Cholesterol/hot water group III (group CH/HW) *"Hot water + Animal diet + Trans-fats"*

The diet taken from the rats in group III (CH/HW) during three weeks was (49.71g±12.94),

(22.30g±3.34) and (29.22g±20.16) respectively. There is a difference in diet consumption between weeks p=0.014.

The Tukey's test indicated that the diet consumed by rats in the second week is decreased significantly when it is compared to the first week p=0.013 (Table07 annex).

Hot water group IV (group HW) *"Hot water + Animal Diet"*

The diet taken from rats in group IV (HW) during the three weeks was (43.64g±5.12),

(45.26g±13.06) and (33.99g±12.32) respectively. There is a difference in diet consumption between weeks p= 0.229.

The Tukey's test indicated that the diet consumed by rats in the third week is decrease not significantly when it is compared to the first week p=0.05 (Table08 annex).

The weight variation

Control group I (group C) *"Normal water + Animal Diet"*

The weight of rats group I (C) during the first, second and third weeks was (103.02g±1.22),

(101.15g±1.80) and (105.09g±2) respectively. There is a difference very highly significantly in weight values between groups of weeks p=0.003.

The Tukey's test indicated that the weight of rats in the third week is increased significantly when it is compared to the second week p=0.002 (table 05 annex).

Cholesterol/water group II (group CH/W) *"Normal water + Animal diet + Trans-fats"*

The weight of rats group (CH/W) during the first, second and the third weeks was (104.36g±3.59), (114.9g±5.59) and (127.88g±1.43) respectively. There is a difference very highly significantly in weight values between weeks p=0.000.

The Tukey's test indicated that the weight of rats in the second week is increased highly significantly when it is compared to the first week p=0.001, and also in the third week is increased highly significantly when it is compared to the first and the second weeks p=0.000 (Table 06 annex).

Cholesterol/hot water group III (group CH/HW) *"Hot water + Animal diet + Trans-fats"*

The weight of rats group (CH/HW) during the first, second and the third weeks was (69.29g±2.48), (79.11g±3.22) and (88.4g±2.15) respectively. There is a difference very highly significantly in weight values between weeks p=0.000.

The Tukey's test indicated that the weight of rats in the second and the third weeks is increased very highly significantly when it is compared to the first week p=0.000, and in the third week is increased very highly significantly when it is compared to the second week p=0.000 (Table 07annex).

Hot water group IV (group HW) *"Hot water + Animal Diet"*

The weight of rats group (HW) during the first, second and the third weeks was (74.86g±1.56) (66.15g±2.20) and (73.38g±3.18) respectively. There is a difference very highly significantly in weight values between weeks p=0.000.

The Tukey's test indicated that the weight of rats in the second week is decreased very highly significantly when it is compared to the first week p= 0.000 and in the third week is increased when it is compared to the second week p=0.000 (Table 08annex).

Results

Water consumption

Control group I (C) *"Normal water + Animal Diet"*

The quantity of water consumed by the rats in group I (C) during the first, second and the third week was (93.83ml±9.67), (116.71ml±14.16) and (117.79ml±50.75) respectively.

There is a difference not significantly in water consumption p=0.395.

The Tukey's test indicated that the water consumed by rats in the third week is increased not significantly when it is compared to the first week p=0.05 (Table09 annex).

Cholesterol/water group II (CH/W) *"Normal water + Animal diet + Trans-fats"*

The consumption of water in group II (CH/W) during the first, second and the third weeks was (104.17ml±8.86), (115.86ml±9.37) and (110.71ml±8.53) respectively. There is a difference not significantly in water consumption p=0.125.

The water consumed by rats in the third week is increased not significantly when it is compared to the first week p=0.05 (Table 09 annex).

Cholesterol/hot water group III (CH/HW) *"Hot water + Animal diet + Trans-fats"*

The consumption of hot water in group III (CH/HW) during the first, second and the third week was (112.50ml±19.53), (80.14ml±6.42) and (70.56ml±10.99) respectively. There is a difference very highly significantly in the water consumption between weeks p=0.000.

The Tukey's test indicated that the water consumed by rats in the second week is decreased highly significantly when it is compared to the first week p= 0.002 and also in the third week is decrease very highly significantly when it is compared to the first week p=0.000 (Table09annex).

Hot water group IV (HW) *"Hot water + Animal Diet"*

The consumption of hot water in group IV (HW) during the first, second and the third week was (126.33ml±25.53), (85ml±21.68) and (90.21ml±9.38) respectively. There is a difference highly significantly in water consumption between weeks p=0.006.

The Tukey's test indicated that the water consumed by rats in the second week is decreased highly significantly when it is compared to the first week p= 0.008 and also in the third week is decreased significantly when it is compared to the first week p=0.020 (Table09annex).

Results

Biochemical results

Lipids status

Total cholesterol

The concentration of total cholesterol was (0.73g±0.10) in group I *"Normal water + Animal Diet,* (0.81g±0.14) in group II *"Normal water + Animal diet + Trans-fats"*, (0.80g±0.03) in group III and (0.89g±0.10) in group IV *"Hot water + Animal Diet"*, our data indicated that the cholesterol is decreased in group III when it is compared to the group II and IV but not significantly p>0.05 (figure 18).

Triglyceride

The concentration of Triglyceride was (0.54g±0.11) in group I *"Normal water + Animal Diet"*, (0.57g±0.17) in group II *"Normal water + Animal diet + Trans-fats"*, (0.44g±0.09) in group III *"Hot water + Animal diet + Trans-fats"* and (0.77g±0.25) in group IV *"Hot water + Animal Diet"*. The Triglyceride concentration was decreased in group III but not significantly when it is compared to the other groups p>0.05 (Figure 19).

HDL-c

The concentration of HDL-c was in group I (0.73g±0.11) *"Normal water + Animal Diet"*, in group II (0.79g±0.15) *"Normal water + Animal diet + Trans-fats"*, in the group III (0.81g±0.07) *"Hot water + Animal diet + Trans-fats"*, and in group IV (0.84g±0.17) *"Hot water + Animal Diet"*. We have observed an increase in the concentration of HDL-c in group III when it is compared to the group I and II, however the concentration of HDL-c in the group IV was higher than the other group but not significantly $p > 0.05$ (Figure 20).

LDL-c

The results of the determination of LDL-c in group I (0.08g±0.01) *"Normal water + Animal Diet"*, group II (0.13g±0.06) *"Normal water + Animal diet + Trans-fats"*, group III (0.10g±0.03) *"Hot water + Animal diet + Trans-fats"* and group IV (0.10g±0.02) *"Hot water + Animal Diet"* showed that there was a difference between groups but not significantly $p > 0.05$ Our data indicated that the LDL-c concentration was decreased in group III and IV treated with hot water when it is compared to the other groups treated with normal water $p > 0.05$ (Figure21).

hs-CRP

The values of hs-CRP were in the group I (0.27g±0.12) *"Normal water + Animal Diet"*, group II (0.66g±0.28) *"Normal water + Animal diet + Trans-fats"*, group III (0.37g±0.12) *"Hot water + Animal diet + Trans-fats"* and group IV (0.7g±0.18) *"Hot water + Animal Diet"*. Our result indicated that the hs-CRP concentration was decreased in group III when it is compared to the groups II and IV but it was slightly higher than group I (Figure22).

Results

1.3. Behavior and morphological investigations

During our study we have noticed that the animals in the group III (CH/HW) *"Hot water + Animal diet + Trans-fats"* are very active when it is compared to other groups. Also we have observed nodules (0.47g, 1.50g and 3.77g) in the neck of three rats in group II (CH/W) *"Normal water + Animal diet + Trans-fats"* and more adipose tissue, otherwise the other groups don't present any nodules and less adipose tissue (photo 01) also we have observed modification on renal color in rat at group II.

1.4. Histological investigation

The weight of organs (liver, heart, aorta, spleen and intestine) in group I *"Normal water + Animal Diet"* was (5.69g, 0.46g, 0.15g,0.51g and 11.65g) respectively. The weight of organs (liver, heart, aorta, spleen and intestine) in group II *"Normal water + Animal diet + Trans-fats"* was (6.14g, 0.55g, 0.17g, 0.64g and 9.79g) respectively. The weight of organs (liver, heart, aorta, spleen and intestine) in group III *"Hot water + Animal diet + Trans-fats"* was (4.70g, 0.40g, 0.15g and 9.33g) respectively. The weight of organs (liver, heart, aorta, spleen and intestine) in group IV *"Hot water + Animal Diet"* was (5.50g, 0.42g, 0.15g and 0.40g) respectively (Figure 27). The organs fixed into the formal solution are kept for future work.

Discussion

Hypercholesterolemia is important in approximately 50 percent of patients with cardiovascular disease, and also it's an indirect factor for the inflammatory bowel disease, other factors need to be taken into consideration. High plasma concentrations of cholesterol, in particular those of low density lipoprotein (LDL) cholesterol, is one of the principal risk factor for atherosclerosis **(Frinklin et al., 2017).**

In this study we have observed that the weight of rats fed with diet rich in Trans-fat and have drink normal water is increased during 21 days of the experimental study. Our result agrees with those of **(Zerizer, 2006)** who reported that an increase in body weight of rats administered with 200 mg/kg of L-methionine during 21 days. However, we have detected that rats diet consumption is decreased during 21 days of the experimental study. Our result is not agrees with those of **(Zerizer, 2006)** who reported that the diet is increased in rats fed with L-methionine during 21 days of experimental study.

Also we have obtained that the weight of rats is increased in group fed with diet rich with

Trans fat and have drink hot water. Our result is agrees with those of **(Zerizer, 2006)** who reported that an increased in body weight of rats administrated with 200 mg/kg of L-methionine and treated with B9 and B12 (0.7mg/kg) and (0.75mg/kg) respectively.

Also we have detected that the quantity of diet consumed by rats is decreased during the experimental study. Our results are not agrees with those of **(Zerizer, 2006)** who reported that the diet consumed by rats fed with L-methionine and treated with vitamin B9 and B12 is increased during 21 days of experimental study.

We could explain that by the influence of hot water on the enzymes which helps the metabolism reaction **(AlHajri, 2010)**.

The increase of levels T-Ch, TG and LDL-c and decrease in HDL-c in rats fed with diet rich with Trans fats. Our result agree with those of **(Deborad et al., 2013)** who reported that, the intake of high levels of saturated fatty acids, Trans fatty acids increase the blood concentration LDL, TG and T-Ch while decreasing the level of HDL. Otherwise, the level of lipids status (T-Ch, TG and LDL-c) are decreased and HDL-c are increased in rats fed with Trans-fats and treated with hot water. This results are in agreement with the work of **(Sakhri, 2014)** who reported that, the lipids status concentration (T-Ch, TG, LDL-c) are decreased and HDL-c concentration increase in mice treated with olive oil.

Also in our study we have confirmed the inflammation process by the increase of hs-CRP in rats fed with trans fats and decreased in rats fed with trans fats and treated with hot water.

This result is agree with those of **(Dorghal and Houadek, 2014)** who reported that the concentration of hs-CRP is decreased in the mice administrated L-methionine and treated with *Vitis vinifera* (500mg/kg) for 12 days.

Our results are in agreement with those of **(AlHajri, 2010)** who reported that hot water dissolve the lipids in our organism and healing the inflammation.

Inflammation in the etiology of vascular events is becoming more obvious as a result of both clinical and laboratory studies. C-reactive protein a non-specific indicator of inflammation, has emerged as a useful parameter for assessing individual risk of cardiovascular disease and acute events. When added to conventional measurements such as cholesterol fractions (LDL and HDL), CRP enhances their discriminatory power **(Scott, 2007).**

We confirmed in this study that the decrease of lipids status and hs-CRP could suppress their cytotoxic effect on the organ tissue by the inhibiting of the tumor formation and adipocyte cells proliferation which due to the inhibitor of pro-inflammatory cytokines.

Otherwise, during our experimental study we detected that the lipids status (T-Ch, TG, LDLc) are increased and the hs-CRP in group of rats fed with animal diet and treated with hot water, this may due to the animal diet alone is poor from vitamins.

Conclusion

In this study we evaluated the relationship between hypercholesterolemia induced by Trans-fats acid with atherosclerosis and inflammatory bowel disease (IBD).

The recommended consumption of hot water play a role on the body weight, and it has an anti-inflammatory effect for long or short term. So the use of hot water seems to have an interest in prevention of atherosclerosis and inflammatory bowel disease (IBD).

The present experimental finding showed that hot water therapy process has a positive effect on the inflammation and a decrease in lipids status.

Based on the present results, our future work and perspectives can evaluate many topics:

➤ We need to keep the water at the same temperature (50°C) for the whole day and night.

➤ Preparation of histological section on different organs (Liver, heart, aorta, sigmoid colon).

➤ Measurement of anti-oxidants, GSH, catalase.

➤ Treatment of animals (rats and mice) with margarine during 21 days or more.

➤ Determination of pro-inflammatory cytokines.

Summary

Cholesterol is a "fat-like" substance present in all body cells, it is a basic component of all cellular membranes and precursor of several hormones, vitamins, and bile acids, and therefore is an essential molecule for life. However, the consumption of saturated and Trans fatty acid is the major causes for the elevation of LDL-c in plasma which is a risk factor for the development of atherosclerosis and inflammatory bowel.

In the present study, we evaluated the benefit of hot water therapy on the inflammation induced by saturated and Trans fats during 21 days in rats, which was evaluated using the detection of hs-CRP and lipids status.

The results showed that the amount of hot water 60-175ml per day for rats could decrease the levels of hs-CRP and lipids status (T-Ch, TG and LDL-c) and increase the concentration of HDL-c.

For this reason, we considered that the hot water is a natural hydrotherapy during short or long term dependent on type of disease.

Benefits of Drinking Hot Water

Therapeutic Methods of Drinking Hot Water (TMDHW) - For Adults

- The recommended consumption of Hot Water shall be at 3 liters daily minimum up to 4 liters maximum.
- Glass, mug or tumbler size - 500 ml, taken in different gulps, not one gulp.
- The maximum consumption of Hot Water shall be 1 liter within One Hour.

Option 1 – Drinking Method for glass size 500 ml

- One to two glasses early in the morning, once you wake up and before brushing your teeth – at standing position (Very important)
- One glass, after brushing your teeth, before having your breakfast.
- One to two glasses throughout the morning.
- One glass 15-30 minutes before lunch. (Very important).
- One to two glasses in the evening.
- One glass, one hour before going to bed (optional.)

Option 2 – Drinking Method for glass size 240-300 ml

- Two glasses of hot water, early in the morning, once you wake up and before brushing your teeth – at standing position – Very important
- One glass of hot water, after brushing your teeth, before having your breakfast (optional).
- Two to three glasses of hot water throughout the morning.
- One glass of hot water at least 15-30 minutes before lunch – Very important.
- Two to three glasses of hot water throughout the evening.
- One glass of hot water, one hour before going to bed.
- The temperature of water shall be around 50oC (122oF), a little bit less than the temperature of hot tea **(AlHajri, 2010).**

Diseases cured in People from drinking hot water therapy

1. Asthma

2. Hypertension (High Blood Pressure)

3. Diabetes Mellitus

4. Migraine & Headache

5. Anemia

6. Series of back pain

7. Urinary Calculus (Stones in the Kidneys)

8. Urinary Tract Infection

9. High Blood Cholesterol

10. Rheumatism & Arthritis

11. Stroke (Cerebral Vascular Accident)

12. Sexual and body weakness

13. Tiredness & Fatigue

14. Tonsillitis

15. Gastroenteritis

16. Insomnia (lack of sleep)

17. Colds, Flu & Fever

18. Heartburn, Ulcer, Constipation (difficulty in passing motion)

19. Parkinsonism (Involuntary Movement of the Body due to old age)

20. Skin Diseases

21. All Kinds of Infections

22. Alzheimer (defects of the Brain)

23. Heart Disease & Heart Abnormality since birth

24. Cancer (there is one case diagnosed and further follow up in other cases is being monitored)

25. Purifying and Regularizing Women's monthly Period (AlHajri, 2010) and (Dhrubo Sen et al., 2015).

References (Chapter 2)

Aaron S B and Andrew P. (2015). The Role of Vitamin D in Inflammatory Bowel Disease.

Healthcare. (3): 338-350.

Alberti S., Schuster G., Parini P., Feltkamp D., Diczfalusy U., Rudling M., Angelin B.,

Björkhem I., Pettersson S., Gustafsson J. (2001). Hepatic cholesterol metabolism and resistance to dietary cholesterol in LXR beta-deficient mice. The Journal of Clinical Investigation. 107(4): 565–573.

Aldons J L. (2000). Atherosclerosis. Nature. 407(6801): 233–241.

AlHajri F. (2010). The miracle & wonders of treatment from hot water: hot water miracles. 1-108.

Alice O., Fred O. (2005). The Role of Cholesterol and Diet in Heart Disease. The Modern Nutritional Diseases. USA. 1-9.

Alzoghaibi M A. (2013). Concepts of oxidative stress and antioxidant defense in Crohn's disease. World J Gastroenterol. 19(39): 6540-6547.

Amit K S., Harsh V S., Arun R., Sanjeev K. (2014). C-reactive protein, inflammation and coronary heart disease. The Egyptian Heart Journal. 67 (2): 89-97.

Anna M J., Debbie F., Sheri Z C. (2016). Nutrition and Health Info Sheet: Trans Fatty Acids. Health Professionals: 1-4.

Anthony C. (2005). LDL Cholesterol: Bad Cholesterol or Bad Science? .Journal of American Physicians and Surgeons. 10(3): 83-89.

Aris P A., Moses E., Haralampos J M. (2011). An overview of lipid abnormalities in patients with inflammatory bowel disease. Annals of Gastroenterology. (24): 181-187.

Barletta C., Luiz E., Raul G. (2004). Johne's disease, Inflammatory Bowel Disease, and Mycobacterium paratuberculosis. Papers in Veterinary and Biomedical Science. 58: 110.

Catherine A O., George T G. (2017). Polygenic Hypercholesterolemia. American Endocrine Society and Mineral Research. Philadelphia. 1-135.

Carol A., Feghali., Timothy M ., Wright M D. (1997). Cytokines in acute and chronic inflammation. Frontiers in Bioscience. 2 (26): 12-26.

Caroline C., Mélanie P., Anne N S., Robert S. (2017). Angiogenesis in the atherosclerotic plaque. Redox Biology. 12: 18–34.

Christian N. (2015). Inflammation: Causes, Symptoms and Treatment. Medical news today. 1-13.

Cortot A. (2003). Crohn's disease. Orphanet Encyclopedia. 1-5.

Crohn's & Colitis Foundation, of America. (2014). Living with Crohn's Disease. Third Avenue. New York. 1-510.

Daniel J R., Jonathan C., Helen H H. (2003). Monogenic hypercholesterolemia: new insights in pathogenesis and treatment. PMC. 111(12): 1795–1803.

Debora E., Claudia M P., Lila M O., Elina B R., Ana R D., Aline D P. (2013). Lipotoxicity: effect of dietary saturated and transfatty acid. Mediators of inflammation. (2013): 1-13.

Donald J., Namara Mc. (2000). Dietary cholesterol and atherosclerosis. Biochemical et Biophysica Acta. 1529 : 310-320.

Dorghal A., Houadek R. (2014). Effet de *Vitis vinifera* sur les maladies inflammatoires chronique de l'intestin (MICI) induites par l'hyperhomocystéinémie. Mémoire présenté en vue de l'obtention du diplôme de magister option : immuno-oncology, Université Mentouri Constantine.

Food and agriculture organization of the United Nations Rome, Fat and fatty acid terminology, methods of analysis and fat digestion and metabolism. Fats and fatty acids in human nutrition-Report of an expert consultation (2010). 22-24

Geetha A., Thiru P N V., Sheela D R., Subramanian S., Kalaiselvi P. (2005). Biochemistry. Tamilnadu. 1-232

George S J., Johnson J. (2010). Atherosclerosis Molecullar and cellular mechanisms. John Wiley & Sons. united kingdom. 1- 420.

Georgia H., Grahaml R., Adford S. (2002). The pathogenesis of Crohn's disease in the 21st century. Pathology. 34 (6): 561-567.

Georgia V., Dimitris T., Christodoulos S H. (2009). The Role of Oxidative Stress in Atherosclerosis. 50: 402-409.

Gerald H T., Daphne O. (2012). LDL as a Cause of atherosclerosis. The Open Atherosclerosis & Thrombosis Journal. 5:13-21.

Gerard J T., Bryan D. (2008). The digestive system. Principles of Anatomy and Physiology. john wiley & sons. 921-924.

Gillman A G., Goodman L S., Rall T W., Murad F. (1985). Lipoprotein. The pharmacological basis of therapeutics. 7th Edition. Macmillan. 1-828.

Guy J. (2008). Differences in Trans Fatty Acids. Health connections. 2(5):2-3

Hanrui Z., Rayan E., Temel., Catherine M. (2014). Cholesterol and lipoprotein metabolism. Arteriosclerosis, Thrombosis and vascular biology. 34:1791-1794.

Isabel D C O., Miguel P., Fernando C. (2013). The fine line between familial and polygenic hypercholesterolemia. Lancet. 381(9874): 1293–1301.

Jagdish K. (2009). Causes, Symptoms, Pathophysiology and diagnosis of atherosclerosis. Pharmacology online. (3): 420-442.

Jana O., Ladislava M., Jarmila VA., Kobert V., Jiri M. Fatty acids composition of vegetable oils and it contribution to dietary energy intake and dependence of cardiovascular mortality on dietary intake of fatty acids. Int Mol Sci.16: 12871-12890.

Jeremy M B., John L T., Lubert S. (2002). The Complex Regulation of Cholesterol Biosynthesis Takes Place at Several Levels. Biochemistry, 5th Edition. New York. 1-1050.

Joseph D F., Adam S C. (2014). Ulcerative Colitis: Epidemiology, Diagnosis, and Management. Mayo Clin Proc. 89(11): 1553-1563.

Kathleen D. (2017). Hyperlipidemia: causes, diagnosis, and treatment. Medical News Today. 2-7.

Kara R. (2010). The Digestive System the human body. Britannica educational publishing. 1-258.

Kim A S., Johnson E R. (2001). Water: Structure and Properties. Encyclopedia of life sciences. 1-7

Leon V., Clark N. (2004). Trends in Atherosclerosis Research. Nova biomedical books. New York. 1- 330.

Lusis A J. (2000). Atherosclerosis. Nature. 407(6801): 233–241.

Manuela M., Martina K., Birgit R., Martin H., Bernhard A. (2004). Hypercholesterolemia in ENU-induced mouse mutants. The Journal of Lipid Research. 45: 2132-2137.

Markus M G. (2015). Cholesterol: Causes and symptoms of high cholesterol. Knowledge center. 1-7.

Masaaki M., Toshio H. (2012). The molecular mechanisms of chronic inflammation development. Frontiers in Immunology. 3(323):1-2.

Mauricio G M., Frank P., Carlos G D. (2014). Cholesterol in brain disease: sometimes determinant and frequently implicated. EMBO reports. 15(10): 1036-1052.

Michael A. (2016). Understanding Inflammation. Johns Hopkins Health review Spring/Summer. 3(1):1-3.

Michael S B., Joseph L. (1995). A Receptor mediated pathway for cholesterol homeostasis. Physiology or medicine. 284-324.

Michael T., Murayn D. (2013). The natural solutions that can change your lif. Cholesterol and heart disease. Canada.1-186.

Mithun J V. (2014). Familial hypercholesterolemia. PMC. 7(2): 107–117.

Moneer F., Nihaya S. (2012). C-Reactive Protein. Blood Cell – An Overview of Studies in Hematology. Baghdad, Iraq. 89-100.

Mooventhan A., Nivethitha L. (2014). Scientific Evidence-Based Effects of Hydrotherapy on Various Systems of the Body. N Am J Med Sci. 6(5): 199–209.

Noah T A., Zachary M W., Randy J N. (2012). Inflammation: Mechanisms,Costs, and Natural Variation. Rev ecol evol Syst. 43:385–406.

Oliver S., Filipe K S. (2013). Trends Hypercholesterolemia links hematopoiesis with atherosclerosis in Endocrinology and Metabolism. 24(3): 129-136.

Ondrejovičová I., Muchová J., Mišľanová C., Nagyová Z., Ďuračková Z. (2010).

Hypercholesterolemia, Oxidative Stress and Gender Dependence in Children. Prague Medical Report . 111(4): 300–312

Paul M. R I., Harles H C., Julie E B., Nader R. (2000). C - reactive protein and other markers of inflammation in production of cardiovascular disease in women. The New England Journal of Medicine. 342 (12).

Pedro M R C., Huanbiao M., Walter J M C., Nirupama S., Andras G L. (2013). The role of cholesterol metabolism and cholesterol transporting carcinogenesis: a review of scientific Findings, relevant to future cancer therapeutics. Frontiers in org. 4(119): 1-7.

Persson PG, Ahlbom A, Hellers G. (1992). Diet and inflammatory bowel disease: a case control study. Epidemiology. 3(1):47-52.

Peter A W., Alex B I., Arch S. (1999). The Acute inflammatory response and it's regulation. 134: 666-669.

Phoebe A S., Adam G G., Milinda E J., Robert W B., Jefferson C F. (2010). Hypercholesterolemia and microvascular dysfunction: interventional strategies. Journal of Inflammation.1-10.

Pirinccioglu A G., Gökalp D., Pirinccioglu M., Kizil G., Kizil M. (2010). Malondialdehyde (MDA) and protein carbonyl (PCO) levels as biomarkers of oxidative stress in subjects with familial hypercholesterolemia. Clin Biochem. 43, 1220–1224. In Ondrejovičová I ., Muchová J ., Mišľanová C ., Nagyová Z ., Ďuračková Z. (2010). Hypercholesterolemia, Oxidative Stress and Gender Dependence in children. Medical Report. 111(4):300–312.

Rafael A C., Mario R., Garcia P. (1990). Cholesterol, Triglycerides, and Associated Lipoproteins. Clinical Methods: The History, Physical, and Laboratory Examinations. 3rd edition. Atlanta, Georgia.1-18.

Raynoo T., Shinji O., Yusuke H., Shiho O., Ning M., Somchai P., Puangrat Y., Shosuke K., Mariko M. (2015). Oxidative stress and its significant roles in neurodegenerative diseases and cancer. int J Mol Sci. (16): 193-217.

Robert H., Nelson MD. (2013). Hyperlipidemia as a Risk Factor for Cardiovascular Disease. Prim Care. 40(1): 195–211.

Rui L Y., Yong H S., Gang H., Wu L., Guo W L. (2008). Increasing the oxidative stress with progressive hyperlipidimia in human: Relation between Malondialdehyde and Atherogenic Index. PMC. 43(3): 154-158.

Ruslan M. (2008). Origin and physiological roles of inflammation. Nature. 454 (10): 1038.

Sakhri F. (2014). Effect of Algerian olive oil on cardiovascular diseases and lipids status in hyperhomocysteinemia treated mice. Thesis submitted for [master's degree]. Option: Biology and molecular physiology, university Constantine 1: 32-34

Severine V., Gert V A., Paul R. (2004). C-reactive Protein as a Marker for Inflammatory Bowel Disease. Inflamm Bowel Dis. 10:661–665.

Scott A., Khan K M., Cook J L. (2004). What is "inflammation"? Are we ready to move beyond Celsius?. Br J Sports Med. 38: 248-249.

Scott J D. (2007). C - reactive protein: An Inflammatory Biomarker in Clinical Practice. The Journal of Lancaster General Hospital. 2 (2): 63-68.

Scoot M., Grundy M D., San D. (1978). Medical Progress Cholesterol Metabolism in Man. West J Med. 128:13-25.

Shakhashiri. (2011). Water. General Chemistry. Chemical of the week. 1-7.

Sheyla L M., Hebeth D P., Maria L P., Renaldo C D S., Eduardo L D O., Marcelo E S 0. (2005). Dietary Models for inducing Hypercholesterolemia in Rats. Brazilian archives of biology and technology. 48(2): 203-209.

Steven B., Irving K., David S. (2004). C - reactive protein. The Journal of Biological Chemistry. 279: 48487-48490.

Stray H C., Chandler A B., Glagov S., Guyton J R., Insull W J., Rosenfeld M E., Schaffer S A., Schwartz C J., Wagner W D., Wissler R W. (1995). Circulation. 92: 1355-1374.

Suluvoy J K. (2017). Protective effect of *Averrhoa bilimbi* fruit extract on ulcerative colitis in wister rats via regulation of inflammatory mediators and cytokines. Biomedicine & Pharmacotherapy. 91:1113–1121.

Taibur R., Ismail H., Towhidul I., Hossain U S. (2012). Oxidative stress and human health. Advances in Bioscience and Biotechnology. 997-1019.

Talmud P J., Shah S., Whittall R. (2013). Use of low-density lipoprotein cholesterol gene score to distinguish patients with polygenic and monogenic hypercholesterolemia: a case– control study. Lancet. 381(9874): 1293–1301.

Tayler F D., Karen M K., Jennifer J M., Raymond W W., Zhihura J. (2009). Lipoproteins, cholesterol homeostasis and cardiac health. Int J Biol Sci. 5 (5):474-488.

Vaclavik V A., Christian E W. (2014). Essentials of Food Science. Food Science. 4th Edition. New York. 1-12.

Volanakis J E. (2001). Human C-reactive protein: expression, structure, and function. Molecular Immunology. 38(2-3): 189–197.

Ward E M. (2008). FATS: Saturated, Polyunsaturated, Monounsaturated, and Trans Fatty acids. Fats.Fact sheet: 1-3.

Wikibooks contributors. (2006). The gastro-intestinal trac. Human physiology. 1-225.

Zerizer S. (2006). Hyperhomocysteinemia, B vitamins and Atherogenesis Clinical and experimental studies. Thesis submitted for the degree of [state doctorate] in natural science. University of Constantine. 33.

Zhang YZ., Li YY. (2014). Inflammatory bowel disease: Pathogenesis. World J Gastroenterology. 20(1): 91-99.

Reference web:

Website. medmovie.com

Crawford MH., DiMarco. (2001). LDL mechanisms oxidation in vessel. Cardiology.

Web site: WebMD Medical Reference from Healthwise

Web site: Johns Hopkins gastroenterology and hepatology

Chapter 3

BRIEF BIOGRAPHY & BRIEF HISTORY

About Faris AlHajri-Ph.D. (A.M.)

Faris AlHajri-Ph.D. (A.M.) is an integrative Nutritional Health Coach, Holistic Health & Wellness international renowned speaker and expert, entrepreneur, researcher, author of two books, discoverer of *Haqua Revitalize*®, and president and founder of Haqua Wellness, Virginia, US.

CREDENTIALS

> ➤ Certified Integrative Health Coach, Institute for Integrative Nutrition, New York, USA (2019)

> ➤ Doctor of Philosophy in Alternative Medicine, Indian Board of Alternative Medicine, India (2013)

> ➤ Independent Holistic Health & Wellness Professional

> ➤ Copyrights held in: USA, Oman, UK & Philippines

> ➤ President, CEO, & Founder: Haqua Wellness, Virginia, USA

> ➤ Expert & Internationally Renowned Speaker on *Haqua Revitalize*® *Therapy – HART*, also known as Hot Water Therapy.

PUBLICATIONS

2-Time Author, Self-published by Authorhouse UK: *The Values of Well-Being & Its Secrets for a Better Living & The Miracle & Wonders of Treatment from Hot Water.*

Book Fairs

- ➢ Book Expo America (New York, NY), 2011.

- ➢ London Book Fair (London, England), 2011.

- ➢ Frankfurt Book Fair (Frankfurt, Germany), 2011.

- ➢ Beijing International Book Fair (Beijing, China), 2011.

- ➢ Muscat 17th International Book Fair (Oman), 2012.

- ➢ Doha 22nd International Book Fair (Qatar), 2011.

Distinctions

- ➢ **Recipient,** Outstanding Excellence to the Scientific Community, San Diego, CA – August 2018.

- ➢ Health Excellence Award 2013, India – March 2013.

- ➢ Recipient of Awards *from one US Congresswoman and two US Senators in honor and recognition of the* My Children's Haven Fundraising Launch *Project and its devotion to the children affected by typhoon Yolanda in July 2016*

Faris AlHajri's Short Bio

Faris AlHajri is an expert and internationally renowned speaker on the exclusively branded *Haqua Revitalize® Therapy – HART* (Aqua Calidum Therapy – ACT, Hydrothermal Therapy – HTT, Hot Aqua Therapy – HAT, Aqua Thermal Therapy – ATT, May Sakhin Therapy – MST, Maji Moto Therapy – MMT, or Hot Water Therapy – HWT). He is a natural born Omani citizen who grew up in Africa, yet was strongly influenced by Western cultures and eventually married a Christian Filipina Nurse and became a father of two energetic sons, Qais and Sami. He proves that love conquers all and neither race nor religion matters when living an authentic life. He was emotionally affected by separation from his mother due to her long-term suffering of health complications, which included undergoing ten surgeries. Unable to achieve his first dream to discover a cure for his mother's 35 years of suffering that ended with uterine cancer that took her life, he sought to discover cures to the ailments of others.

First a Quantity Surveyor by profession that included various government positions, he labored intensively to both provide and bury himself in a distraction from the pain he felt at the loss of his mother until he, too, developed various health complications. As his health deteriorated, despite his best efforts to maintain health including proper nutrition, his two young children became concerned and a cloud of despair started to fill his home. Failure was no longer an option, so he intensified his efforts to find a permanent cure for his advanced chronic attacks of bronchial asthma, lower backache (Lumbago), migraines and allergic rhinitis. The result of his efforts was the physical, mental and spiritual health cure of *Haqua Revitalize® Therapy – HART* and *Amplify Your Subconscious Vitality*.

Faris also involved his family in participating in and reaping the benefits of using *Haqua Revitalize® Therapy*. He claims that as a result of HART, both he and his family have become completely asymptomatic, and from August 2007 through present time, he and his family members have not taken any other medication. The HART practitioner believes that water is the elixir of our life and can be harnessed to cure many ailments. Faris desires to promote healthy living and has thereby devoted his life completely to help spread natural health and wellness awareness. He has travelled the globe extensively to speak at international conferences, conduct workshops and seminars on this topic, and has written two books: *The Miracle & Wonders of Treatment from Hot Water* and *The Values of Well Being & Its Secrets for a Better Living - Theories*. His goal is to help every individual by spreading awareness of the importance of the miraculous benefits of *Haqua Revitalize® Therapy*, and its concealed scientific mysteries never before revealed.

Since his discovery in August 2007 through today, Faris and his family members have been deeply immersed in practicing BICADU Principles (Believe, Implement, Continue, Appreciate, Discipline, and Understand) of HART. Faris has sought to extend his discovery to every individual who seeks to live an entirely healthy lifestyle by practicing all PEMS Aspects of Health (Physical, Emotional, Mental, and Spiritual), and facilitates spreading his knowledge via conducting speeches at international conferences, lectures and seminars, direct coaching, a strong social media presence, and providing assistance to any individual seeking to achieve ultimate healthy living.

With his lifelong ambitions accomplished, he now devotes himself completely to intensifying research in support of his scientific discovery. He received his Doctorate of Philosophy in Alternative Medicines from the Indian Board of Alternative Medicine (IBAM), approved by the Open International University. Faris desires to promote healthy living and has devoted his life completely to spreading the awareness of natural health & wellness by facilitating understanding the importance of the miraculous benefits of *Haqua Revitalize® Therapy*.

Faris is internationally well-travelled and spends a significant portion of his time researching and postulating ideas. Overwhelmed by the beauty of nature, he strongly believes our world of miracles holds direct and indirect benefits, and sincerely appreciates every human's worth. He desires for a simple and peaceful environment and crusades to promote understanding and forgive wrongdoing. He strives to be a virtual representation of a calm, centered person who practices emotional self-control in every situation. He has adopted the basic principle in life that all human beings share common factors of unity between them, and their differences are for the sake of sharing what could never be found from oneself. He fully embodies advocacy of peace with the intention of sharing his knowledge through his books of wellness.

MEMBERSHIPS & AFFILIATIONS

- ➤ Editorial Member, ACTA Scientific Neurology (India), since Feb. 2019.

- ➤ Member, American Association for the Advancement in Science (USA), since 2017.

- ➤ Member, Philippine College for the Advancement in Medicine (Philippines), Lifetime.

- ➤ Member, Islamic Psychology Conference (United Arab Emirates), Lifetime.

- ➤ Board of Directors, My Children's Haven Org (USA), 2016-2017.

- ➤ Member, Academy of Integrative Health & Medicine (USA), 2015-2017.

- ➤ Honorary Advisor, World Yoga Foundation, (India), 2015-2020.

- ➤ Honorary Patron, Sandhya Maarga Holistic Living Academy (Malaysia), 2015-2020.

- ➤ Member, American Holistic Health Association (AHHA) (USA), since 2014.

- ➤ Member, Oman American Business Center (Oman), since 2014.

Events

- ➤ Organizing committee member, speaker, and chair at eight International Conferences in San Diego, US; Melbourne, Australia; Kolkata, India; Manila, Philippines; Abu Dhabi, Dubai; and Sharjah, UAE.

- ➤ Interviewed & Featured in 92 Media, Live TV, Radios, Magazines, Newspapers & Press Releases in US, UK, Oman, UAE, Qatar, Philippines, Malaysia, and Saudi Arabia.

- ➤ Published Three Peer Reviewed Articles.

- ➤ Conducted 60 Seminars, Workshops, and Lectures at Universities, Colleges, Health Organizations, Schools, and Public and Private Organizations in Oman, UAE, Philippines, and US.

- ➤ Conducted Training, Technical aspects of the Administrative & Financial Affairs activities- Muscat.

About Haqua Wellness & Its Vision

Haqua Wellness, Blacksburg, Virginia is an organization dedicated to promoting healthy, holistic healing through *Haqua Revitalize® Therapy (HART)*. The business plan is to operate as a holistic health spa providing individual treatment, engage in online and live education, actively collaborate with universities and other health & wellness practitioners to study the benefits of *Haqua Revitalize® Therapy*, and to continue to publish and promote Dr. AlHajri's international work in this area of holistic health. The vision is to establish proposed Haqua Wellness Resort & Spa (HAWERS), Haqua Wellness Center (HAWEC), Haqua Global Wellness City (HAGlOWEC), Haqua Wellness Organization non-profit (HWO), and even more wellness projects.

About Professor Zerizer

Professor and director of research at Université Les Frères Mentouri, Constantine, Algeria. Zerizer S. earned a Master's degree from University of Salford, Manchester, England in 1987 Department of Biochemistry, and completed PhD in 2006 from Faculty of Natural Sciences, University of Frères Mentouri, Constantine, Algeria.

About the Students Thesis for their Master Degree

Country	: **People's Democratic Republic of Algeria**
Government Body	: Ministry of Higher Education and Scientific Research
Academy	: University of Frères Mentouri Constantine
Faculty	: Life and Natural Sciences
Department	: Animal Biology
Purpose of the Study	: Thesis submitted by a group of students for their Master's Degree
Option	: Immuno-oncology
Study name	: The Effect of hot water on inflammation induced by hypercholesterolemia in rats
Presented by	: Guennoub Sabrina and Redouane Ali Rachida
Date presented (day/month/year)	: 13/07/2017
Examination Board	
Chairman	: Dr. Messoudi S. (MAA – UFM Constantine)
Supervisor	: Pr. Zerizer S. (Prof. - UFM Constantine).
Examiner	: Dr. Aribi B. (MAB-UFM Constantine).

The History behind the Clinical Study

From the day we discovered that a change in water's temperature would be the secret key to not only treating or preventing ailments, including chronic ones, but also revitalizing the entire human body back to its state of physical, emotional, mental, and spiritual healthy lifestyle; we never hesitated sharing to the public, regardless of race, age, ancestry, color, disability (mental and physical), gender expression, gender identity, genetic information, marital status, medical condition, military or veteran status, national origin, political affiliation, religious creed, sexual orientation, citizenship status, religion, or identity. We also entirely refused to get paid while bringing the awareness to the public, conducting speeches at local and international conferences, interviews with the media, conducting lectures and seminars in universities, colleges, elementary and high schools, churches, mosques, public and private organizations, etc. We maintained our personal philosophy of avoiding asking anyone's denominations, not even their races, gender, or physical, financial, or political affiliations.

It all started on the day back in March 2017 when I received an email from Professor Zerizer saying as follows:

"I have seen your video about the treatment with hot water last January where I was looking for deficiency of vitamin D3. So since that time I started drinking hot water also I had stress hypertension so now I am waiting to do blood analysis for the vitamin D3 and I will see the effect of hot water on this vitamin for the hypertension until now I feel better, meanwhile I eat healthy food. Actually I will start a research work with my master students so I decided to use hot water as treatment for inflammation on the rats administered with high concentration of saturated fatty acid or methionine. So please my question is; do you think I can do this experiment or not?"

We then replied with our optimistic view as follows: "First, I am delighted for you interest to conduct a research work with your master students using Hot Water as a treatment for inflammation on the rats administered with high concentration of saturated fatty acid or methionine. Secondly, yes, I would strongly recommend you to do the proposed research. We do request for a working relation to advise the researchers on protocols and other implementation methods. As for the research itself, a little research on the rats' metabolism and the temperature of their systems I think."

Meanwhile Prof. Zerizer was interested in implementing the hot water protocol in herself, which we highly recommended to her, and sent to her the therapeutic methods of drinking hot water. She later sent us her medical checkups, which have shown her vitamin D deficiency had improved and her blood pressure at a sport club was 14.7/8, then she drunk hot water when she returned home and it decreased to 9.9/6. But she was concerned because her body weight decreased from 60.5kg to 58.4kg.

We then provided her some health guidance, including, but not limited to the following:

"Regarding your concern in losing weight, let me explain you here in brief; (a) Hot Water Therapy helps losing weight, due to fact it melt the fat deposits (speeding up the reaction of enzymes in breaking down the substances (fats to fatty acids, carbohydrates to glucose, proteins to amino acids) and again breaking them down to produce energy for the cells and building and strengthening the muscles. (b) Calorie is directly linked to water and heat, hot water naturally is the secret key to calorie burning and uniquely by hydration, without even any physical activities. The last is hence for additional benefits, but not the prime cause of losing weight. (c) Hot water therapy helps naturally producing vitamin D through the cholesterol sulfate under the skin, the cholesterol in the blood vessels leave to fill up the cholesterol sulfate. The cholesterol plaque leaves the wall of the blood vessels, and cholesterol is hereby controlled. A great news for prevention of high cholesterol, high blood pressure, heart disease, diabetes, etc. (d) hot water therapy leads to vasodilation - an increase to blood veins- by thermogenesis. A great news for the blood to properly distribute vitamins, proteins, oxygen, hydrogen, energy to the body's cells. More and more health benefits, may not be possible to cover them all under a short message. Thus, weight loss would be a normal reaction, and within time, of continuing the hot water therapy regularly as per the daily program, would lead to increase of the periosteum - the bone density- which would help regulating the body's weight and body fitness."

We then emphasized to her to keep to the Hot Water therapy, mostly with the Therapeutic Methods of Drinking Hot Water (TMDHW) in addition to the Hydrothermal Towel Therapy (HTTT), to speed up the reaction of the cholesterol under the skin to naturally increase her Vitamin D production.

As prof. Zerizer kept sending her medical checkups for her vitamin D deficiency and her improvement with the hot water therapy, we then prepared and sent her a health report below which covered her answer to our inquiries as well, as follow:

Table 01: Dr. Zerizer's concentrations of Vitamin D3 before and after drinking hot water.

Date (d/m/y)	2/10/2016	12/01/2017	06/02/2017	18 /03/2017	28/03/2017	8/04/2017
Level of Vitamin D	11ng/ml	8.9 ng/ml	41.6 ng/ml	27.1 ng/ml	15.18 ng/ml	26.3 ng/ml
Note	Before having hot water	Started drinking hot water & had one dose of vitamin D3	Having hot water	Having hot water	Having hot water	Having hot water
Location	At Algeria Lab	At Algeria Lab	At Algeria Lab	At Algeria Lab	Tunisia Lab	At Algeria Lab

Observation:

On 12/01/2017 (day/month/year), she had one dose only of Vitamin D3 of 200,000UI/1ml, and she has been drinking hot water from 12/01/2017 until now.

In Algeria's lab, the concentration of vitamin D3 was 27.1 ng/ml and she repeated the dosage of Vitamin D3 in Tunisia Laboratory, she found that the concentration was 15.18 ng/ml so when she returned back home she repeated again the dosage it was 26.3 ng/ml.

Prof. Zerizer then reported that she was thinking about why the level of vitamin D3 had decreased to 15 ng/ml, and realized that the quantity of hot water which she had consumed in Tunisia was lower than when she was at home.

Notes/ Inquiries on Personal Research:

Sr.	Questions by Faris AlHajri	Answers by Prof. Zerizer
	First Column: Is the date supposed to be 2/10/2016?	Sorry I [made a] mistake. Yes, it is 2/10/2016.
	Is the one dose of Vitamin D3 done once only throughout the test? If not, how frequently, or how did you spread the dosage?	The doctor gave me 3 doses of vitamin D3 for three months and I [drank] only one dose in 12/01/2017 before seeing your video about hot water.
	Is the dosage 200,000 UI/ml? or 200 UI/ml? (The first would be too high, and the second would be too low, please clarify exactly)	The first one (200 000 UI/ml) even when I have seen the doctor in Tunisia, he gave me three doses of vitamin D3 every 15 days I should have one dose of 200,000 UI/ml.
	When you said you repeated the dosage, when did this happen? Did you repeat the dosage right before the measurement or earlier? Or when you said repeated the dosage, you mean the tests?	I did the last dosage of vitamin D3 before going to Tunisia and after returning home the [dates] are mentioned in the table, I found that there is a difference in the concentration of vitamin D3; this is due to maybe the method and reagent used in the analysis.
	Did you take in the dosage of Vitamin D3 before hot water also and tested results without the hot water therapy? That way we can differentiate between hot water therapy and without hot water therapy.	Yes of course I mentioned that in the table before and after I found that there is a difference in the concentration.

	Where did you test the last/ highest concentration of Vitamin D3?	I did the last test in Algeria.
	Do you have an explanation to the decrease in the concentration when you went to Tunisia Laboratory?	Maybe due to different [methods] and [reagents] used for the analysis but usually during the research when we repeat the analysis for any parameter we found only small [differences], not as I have.
	Do you have written reports for the tests that you conducted?	Yes I will send them to you
	Would you kindly re-arrange the Table 01 vitamin D3, in serial manner, by time, from earlier to latest time recorded, and send it back to me again after correction, including correction of the date as mentioned in item (1) above?	Yes ok

Case Report

In conclusion, it's been observed that there was a good improvement in Dr. Zerizer's Vitamin D deficiency.

On Oct. 2, 2016, before starting the hot water therapy, the Vitamin D3 level was extremely low at 11ng/ml. This is considered severely deficient.

Vitamin deficiency could lead to Osteomalacia. Characteristics of this disease are softening of the bones, leading to bending of the spine, bowing of the legs, proximal muscle weakness (muscles closest to the body's midline), bone fragility, and increased risk for fractures. [1, 4]

Osteomalacia reduces calcium absorption and increases calcium loss from bone, which increases the risk for bone fractures. Osteomalacia is usually present when 25-hydroxyvitamin D levels are less than about 10 ng/mL. [1, 5] Low blood levels of vitamin D are associated with increased mortality,[1, 2] as well as some cancers, increased risk of viral infections, tuberculosis, multiple sclerosis, gestational diabetes, bowing of the legs, softening of the bones, muscle weakness, bone fragility, and increased risk for fractures. [1, 3]

In April 8, 2017 (final test), there was a dramatic improvement on the level of Vitamin D3, reaching to 26.3 ng/ml, despite the difference in Algeria and Tunisia Labs, but at least it has improved without taking any vitamin supplements (except the first dosage, as shown in Table 01 above). This result was generally considered adequate for bone and overall health in healthy individuals, as shown on the following table.

In January 12, 2017, as earlier emphasized, having taken one dose of Vitamin D3 of 200 000UI/1ml, this was observed to be very high. We advised Prof. Zerizer that it was good she had taken her decision to stop further doses, otherwise it could have led to vitamin toxicity. In healthy adults, sustained intake of more than 1250 µg/day (micrograms/day, 50,000 IU (International Units)) can produce overt toxicity after several months and can increase serum 25-hydroxyvitamin D levels to 150 ng/ml and greater.[1, 6, 7] Those with certain medical conditions are far more sensitive to vitamin D and can develop hypercalcemia—high calcium (Ca^{2+}) levels in the blood serum—in response to any increase in vitamin D nutrition.[1, 8, 9] Vitamin D toxicity is treated by discontinuing vitamin D supplementation and restricting calcium intake. Kidney damage may be irreversible. [1, 8]

The following table showed Prof. Zerizer's health status:

Table 02: Serum 25-Hydroxyvitamin D [25(OH)D] Concentrations and Health. [10, 11]

nmol/L	ng/mL	Health status
<30	<12	Associated with vitamin D deficiency, leading to rickets in infants and children and osteomalacia in adults
30 to <50	12 to <20	Generally considered inadequate for bone and overall health in healthy individuals
≥50	≥20	Generally considered adequate for bone and overall health in healthy individuals
>125	>50	Emerging evidence links potential adverse effects to such high levels, particularly >150 nmol/L (>60 ng/mL)

We finally sent her a glimpse on Hot Water Therapy with regards to Vitamin D:

Hot Aqua Therapy (both the TMDHW-Therapeutic Methods of Drinking Hot Water, and the HTTT-Hydrothermal Towel Therapy) is highly effective to the body, which has its own innate ability to produce vitamin D, and could eliminate the discrepancy in regards to the danger of vitamin D toxicity from those obtained by supplements.

Sunlight is a natural source of vitamin D on our skin, helping our body to deposit calcium in the bones. This is due to the heat being produced by the sun; in turn, the body receives energy from the sun. Hot Water Therapies could provide the same effects, without causing any harm. Abiding the Hot Aqua Therapy, along with just a few minutes of sunbathing, body exercising and proper nutrition, would be highly suggested to attain similar benefits of the sun, but in addition to hydration of the cells.

In November 2017, Prof. Zerizer informed us that she needed us to see the results of Master thesis. Meanwhile she needed answers to another question, which came as follows:

"On the effect of hot water on trans fats, I found that the group of animals treated with hot water and feed with aliment rich in trans fats that the concentration of the lipids status are decreased when it is compared to the control group and experimental group feed with trans fats and normal water but the positive group the rats feed with normal aliment and hot water we found that the lipid status (T-cholesterol, Triglyceride LDL- cholesterol) and the hs-CRP are increased however the HDL-cholesterol is decreased and the rats were tired and some of them are ill. SO I concluded that during drinking hot water we need to eat Trans fats and fats but if we eat aliments poor in lipids and drinking hot water that we could feel tired and we lose weight and we can dying. SO I need your opinion about that. Also during your conferences you demonstrated that the hot water kills the harmful bacteria so my question is how hot water could distinguish between harmful bacteria and good bacteria because when we drink 3liters per day hot water could kills all good bacteria."

Below are Prof. Zerizer's comments and our answers accordingly as follow;

Sr.	Comments by Prof. Zerizer	Answers by Faris AlHajri
1	On the effect of hot water on trans fats I found that the group of animals treated with hot water and feed with aliment rich in trans fats that the concentration of the lipids status are decreased when it is compared to the control group and experimental group feed with trans fats and normal water but the positive group the rats feed with normal aliment and hot water we found that the lipid status (T-cholesterol, Triglyceride, LDL-cholesterol) and the hs-CRP are increased however the HDL-cholesterol is decreased and the rats were tired and some of them are ill	Hot Water Therapy doesn't only reduce lipid concentration, but it regulates it. Thus, in review to your experiment with rats, it is clear that when the rats were treated with hot water and fed with aliment rich in trans fats the concentration of the lipids status decreased, due to the fact, to prevent any excessive lipid concentration in the blood veins, the liver, etc. Whereas, in the occurrence where the rats were fed with normal aliment and hot water, the lipid status (T-cholesterol, Triglyceride, LDL-cholesterol) and the hs-CRP are increased, as to maintain the amount of lipids concentration the body requires, otherwise, if there is a continuous reduction in lipid concentration, then there would definitely lead to some health complications within time, even in the occurrence of HDL-cholesterol is decreased, this would also get regulated to the normal range.

2	The rats were tired and some of them are ill.	I am very certain the rats were not ill, but, due to the detoxification method the rats have been going through, and as the result from the hot water therapy, it is always normal to occur such incident. This symptom, is typical to after practicing body exercise or workouts, of after having been undergoing massage therapy, of a spa of Hot Bath Method, etc. As the body undergo a complete relaxation and may need some rest. Nothing to worry about this at all. You are advised to continue your experimentation to the rats and see the results afterwards.
3	I concluded that during drinking hot water we need to eat trans fats and fats but if we eat aliments poor in lipids and drinking hot water that we could Feel tired and we lose weight and we can dying	We have conducted a research on Hot Aqua Therapy and Nutrition. This is a complete new type of dieting, where we recommend cutting down food intake by 50-70%, and up to 90%, on daily basis, and substitute it with the Hot Water Therapy. The person is then trained to undergo through the "Body's Manifestation". That is, eating whatever the body may crave, at a lower volume, and eat as much the body would crave, once weekly. Meal times "Breakfast, lunches, and dinners" are becoming unnecessary, and the person would have to eat only when he or she craves for food, again, at a lower volume as mentioned. - According to the Tenets of Osteopathy, the body's innate ability for self-healing, self-protection, and self-regulation. In addition, the lipid under the skin produces cholesterol sulfate (as discovered by an American Scientist, Dr. Stephanie Seneff, a senior research scientist at the Massachusetts Inst. of Technology). The lipid in the blood veins leave to fill up the lipid under the skin. Hot Water Therapy keeps maintaining this cycle frequently, as the person abides with the Therapeutic Methods of Drinking Hot Water regularly.

		- On the issue of losing weight, yes, there is a direct correlation between calorie burning and Hot Water. As to the definition of calorie, it is the energy our body needs, while raising the temperature of one gram water from 14.5 to 15.5 degree Celsius. That doesn't mean, as the person maintain the daily recommended Methods of Drinking Hot Water, will keep losing weight, rather, the body weight will be regulated at a constant level. Due to the fact that, as the body keeps burning calories and losing weight, in the meantime, the calcium concentration will remain stronger, and the bones will maintain its minerals, and proteins to keep it strong and dense. So, it is a cycle the body goes through, to maintain its fitness. Neither fatty, nor skinny.
4	During your conferences you demonstrated that the hot water kills the harmful bacteria so my question is how could hot water distinguish between harmful bacteria and good bacteria because when we drink 3 liters per day hot water could kills all good bacteria.	In 1877, two researchers, Downes and Blunt, discovered that sunlight can destroy harmful bacteria. The fact is that sunlight produces energy the body needs, and the heat produced can only destroy harmful bacteria, and not the good ones. This is one of the hidden mysteries of the power of nature. Hot Water Therapy maintains the amount of energy the body needs frequently, and would destroy harmful bacteria in the body, not the good ones.

| 5 | | In conclusion to all above, I would like to inform you that, I myself, and many thousands of our followers, have been strictly abiding with the daily Therapeutic Methods of Drinking Hot Water, in addition to its other modalities, since we discovered it in August 2007, until the present time. You may take a quick look in one of our follower testimonials, in our You Tube channel, through our website below. We have been maintaining a perfect healthy condition for the last ten years. Since then, no one of my entire family members (including my wife) have ever taken any single medication. This is for your knowledge. |

References (Chapter 3)

1. Vitamin D. Wikipedia, the free encyclopedia. http://en.wikipedia.org/wiki/Vitamin_D - accessed December 19, 2013

2. "Rickets".http://www.nhs.uk/conditions/Rickets/Pages/Introduction.aspx. National Health Service. March 8, 2012. Retrieved July 9, 2012.

3. Avenell A, Mak JC, O'Connell D (April 2014). "Vitamin D and vitamin D analogues for preventing fractures in post-menopausal women and older men". The Cochrane Database of Systematic Reviews. 4 (4): CD000227. doi:10.1002/14651858.CD000227.pub4. PMID 24729336.

4. Insel, Paul; Ross, Don; Bernstein, Melissa; Kimberley McMahon (18 March 2015). Discovering Nutrition. Jones & Bartlett Publishers. ISBN 978-1-284-06465-0

5. Holick MF (March 2006). "High prevalence of vitamin D inadequacy and implications for health". Mayo Clinic Proceedings. **81** (3): 353–73. doi:10.4065/81.3.353. https://www.ncbi.nlm.nih.gov/pubmed/16529140.

6. Holick MF (July 2007). "Vitamin D deficiency". The New England Journal of Medicine. 357 (3): 266–81. doi:10.1056/NEJMra070553. https://www.ncbi.nlm.nih.gov/pubmed/17634462

7. Vitamin D at Merck Manual of Diagnosis and Therapy Professional Edition. http://www.merck.com/mmpe/sec01/ch004/ch004k.html.

8. Vieth R (May 1999). "Vitamin D supplementation, 25-hydroxyvitamin D concentrations, and safety" (PDF). http://www.ajcn.org/content/69/5/842.full.pdf. The American Journal of Clinical Nutrition. 69 (5): 842–56. https://www.ncbi.nlm.nih.gov/pubmed/10232622.

9. Tolerable Upper Intake Limits for Vitamins And Minerals (PDF). http://www.efsa.europa.eu/en/home/oldsc/upper_level_opinions_full-part33.pdf. European Food Safety Authority. December 2006. ISBN 92-9199-014-0.

10. Vitamin D. National Institute of Health. https://ods.od.nih.gov/factsheets/VitaminD-HealthProfessional/#en1 accessed May 17, 2017.

11. Institute of Medicine, Food and Nutrition Board. Dietary Reference Intakes for Calcium and Vitamin D. Washington, DC: National Academy Press, 2010.

Chapter 4

COVID-19 & HAQUA REVITALIZE THERAPY-HART

(PP Presentation-for a quick review)

COVID-19 & Haqua Revitalize Therapy-HART

Faris AlHajri - PhD(AM)
Haqua Wellness - Blacksburg, VA
AlHajri Holistic Health & Wellness LLC - VA, USA

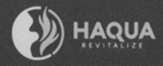

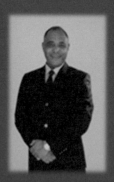

Since 2007

Copyrights: US, UK, Oman, & Philippines

COVID-19 & *Haqua Revitalize® Therapy (HART)*

A brief about COVID-19

The coronavirus disease 2019 (COVID-19), which used to be called the novel coronavirus (2019-nCoV), is a new type of coronavirus that causes respiratory illness in people. It was first identified in Wuhan, China. COVID-19 can spread from person to person. [1]

COVID-19 & Haqua Revitalize® Therapy (HART)

COVID-19 - Symptoms

Begin 2-14 days after you get infected. They include:
- Fever
- Cough
- Shortness of breath

Most of the people infected have pneumonia in both lungs.[1]

COVID-19 & Haqua Revitalize® Therapy (HART)

COVID-19 - Outbreak

As of 27 February 2020, there have been

2,810 confirmed deaths and more than

82,500 confirmed cases in the

coronavirus (COVID-19) outbreak.[2,3,4]

COVID-19 & Haqua Revitalize® Therapy (HART)

Because this is a new virus, there are still things we do not know, such as how severe the illness can be, how well it is transmitted between people, and other features of the virus. (Minnesota Dept. of Health)[5]

COVID-19 & Haqua Revitalize® Therapy (HART)

The new coronavirus attacks the lungs, and in about 20% of patients, infections can become more serious. As the virus enters lung cells, it starts to replicate, destroying the cells, explains Dr. Yoko Furuya, an infectious disease specialist at Columbia University Irving Medical Center.[6]

COVID-19 & Haqua Revitalize® Therapy (HART)

The immune system response to this invader can also destroy lung tissue and cause inflammation. The end result can be pneumonia. That means the air sacs in the lungs become inflamed and filled with fluid, making it harder to breathe. (Dr. Yoko Furuya) [6]

COVID-19 & Haqua Revitalize® Therapy (HART)

The symptoms can also make it harder for the lungs to get oxygen to your blood, potentially triggering a cascade of problems. "The lack of oxygen leads to more inflammation, more problems in the body. Organs need oxygen to function, right? So when you don't have oxygen there, then your liver dies and your kidney dies," says Dr. Carlos del Rio, a professor of medicine and global health at Emory University [6]

COVID-19 & Haqua Revitalize® Therapy (HART)

That's what seems to be happening in the most severe cases. About 3% to 5% of patients end up in intensive care, according to the WHO. And many hospitalized patients require supplemental oxygen. (Dr. Yoko Furuya)[6]

COVID-19 & Haqua Revitalize® Therapy (HART)

People with other underlying medical conditions, such as heart disease, diabetes or chronic lung disease, have also proved most vulnerable. Those kinds of conditions can make it harder for the body to recover from infections. (Dr. Yoko Furuya)[6]

COVID-19 & Haqua Revitalize® Therapy (HART)

During infection of the coronavirus COVID-19, high levels of inflammatory cytokines have been reported.[7]
Cytokines are small secreted proteins released by cells that have a specific effect on the interactions and communications between cells. Cytokines act in concert with specific cytokine inhibitors and soluble cytokine receptors to regulate the human immune response.[8]

COVID-19 & Haqua Revitalize® Therapy (HART)

When liver cells are inflamed or damaged, they can leak higher than normal amounts of enzymes into the bloodstream. One recent report (published in the *Lancet Journals*) found signs of liver damage in a person with COVID-19. Doctors says it's not clear, though, if the virus or the drugs being used to treat the person caused the damage. [9]

COVID-19 & Haqua Revitalize® Therapy (HART)

With any infection, the body's immune system responds by attacking the foreign virus or bacteria. While this immune response can rid the body of the infection, it can also sometimes cause collateral damage in the body. [9]

COVID-19 & Haqua Revitalize® Therapy (HART)

This can come in the form of an intense inflammatory response, sometimes called a "cytokine storm." The immune cells produce cytokines to fight infection, but if too many are released, it can cause problems in the body. [9]

COVID-19 & Haqua Revitalize® Therapy (HART)

How may Haqua Revitalize Therapy® help
treating Coronavirus (COVID-19)?

Future of Medicine
Notable Doctors Perspective!

 HAQUA

COVID-19 & Haqua Revitalize® Therapy (HART)

Personal Perception

" The FEELs (Four Essential Elements of Life) are
the human's body essential fuels, which revitalize the
body to maintain its PEMS (physical, emotional,
mental, and spiritual) innate potentials towards self-
healing, self-regulation and self-maintenance."

~ Faris AlHajri-Ph.D.(A.M.)

 HAQUA

COVID-19 & Haqua Revitalize® Therapy (HART)

Haquate means to make the body absorb the Four Essential Elements of Life (FEELs); namely, water, oxygen, hydrogen and energy (WOHE).
Haquate derives from "Haqua."

"Haqua Revitalize®" is the reinstatement of the human's body to its initial state of creation in the precise form of complete physical, emotional, mental, and spiritual (PEMS) aspects of health.

COVID-19 & Haqua Revitalize® Therapy (HART)

Among the three tenets of Osteopathic Medicine, which express the underlying philosophy of osteopathic medicine, are: the body is capable of self-regulation, self-healing, and health maintenance. (American Osteopathic Association) [10]

The human body's immune system would gradually start crumpling the moment it is depleted from one or more of its essential fuels, the FEELs.

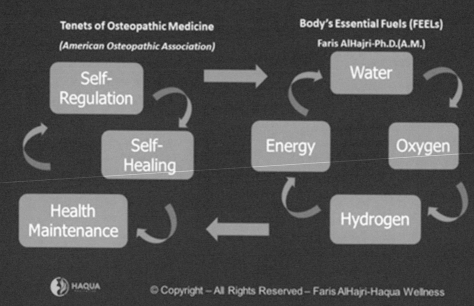

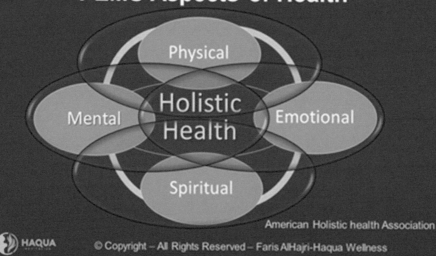

COVID-19 & Haqua Revitalize® Therapy (HART)

4 Essential Elements of Life (FEELs)
(Body's Essential Fuels)

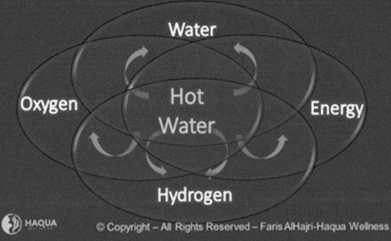

COVID-19 & Haqua Revitalize® Therapy (HART)

A 2017 thesis submitted by a group of students for the degree of Master of Immuno-oncology from the University of Frères Mentouri Constantine in Algeria, on the effects of hot water on inflammation induced by hypercholesterolemia in rats, by conducting a peer-review of Faris AlHajri's recommended consumption of hot water, concluded as follows: [11]

COVID-19 & Haqua Revitalize® Therapy (HART)

University of Frères Mentouri Constantine, Algeria

The effects of hot water on inflammation induced by hypercholesterolemia in rats

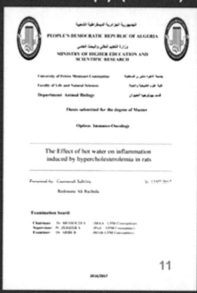

11

COVID-19 & Haqua Revitalize® Therapy (HART)

Introduction (part)

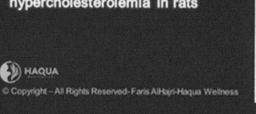

The use of water for various treatments (hydrotherapy) is probably as old as mankind.

Hydrotherapy is one of the basic methods of treatment widely used in the system of natural

medicine, which is also called as water therapy.

11

COVID-19 & Haqua Revitalize® Therapy (HART)

Hot Water purifies the toxin, helps melting the fat deposits and destroys harmful bacteria in our body. It is the most important catalyst in losing weight, it can also help the gastrointestinal tract to function even better. It's get rid of fat, reduce obesity, and cured high blood cholesterol, Stroke, Gastroenterisis, Heart Disease (**Alhajri, 2010**).

Objectives

- Evaluate the effect of saturated, Trans fatty acids and hot water on the weight and diet of rats.

- Evaluate the effect of hot water on hypercholesterolemia induced by Trans fats by measuring the levels of T-Ch, HDL-c, LDL-c and TG.

- Evaluate the effect of hot water on the inflammation by measuring C-reactive protein induced by hypercholesterolemia.

11

COVID-19 & Haqua Revitalize® Therapy (HART)
Inflammatory disease (part)

IV. INFLAMMATION

IV.1. DEFINITION

The word inflammation comes from the Latin *"inflammo"*, meaning *"I set alight, I ignite »*, or inflammare (to set on fire) (**Christian, 2015**) and (**Scott, 2004**). Inflammation underlies a wide variety of physiological and pathological processes (**Ruslan, 2008**). It is a biological reaction to a disrupted tissue homeostasis (**Noah et al., 2012**). It is the body's attempt at self protection, the aim being to remove harmful stimuli, including damaged cells, irritants, or pathogen and begin the healing process (**Christian, 2015**).

Inflammation is critical for the development of many complex diseases and disorders including autoimmune diseases, metabolic syndrome, neurodegenerative diseases, cancers, and cardiovascular diseases (**Masaaki and Toshio, 2012**).

11

COVID-19 & Haqua Revitalize® Therapy (HART)

IV.2. TYPES OF INFLAMMATION

IV.2.1. Acute inflammation

The acute inflammation is characterized by increased blood flow and vascular permeability along with the accumulation of fluid, leukocytes, and inflammatory mediators such as cytokine (**Carol et al., 1997**). It is starts rapidly and quickly and becomes severe. The Signs and symptoms are only present for a few days, but in some cases may persist for a few weeks (**Christian, 2015**).

IV.2.2. Chronic inflammation

Chronic inflammation is characterized by the development of specific humoral and cellular immune responses to the pathogen(s) present at the site of tissue injury (**Carol et al., 1997**). This means long-term inflammation, which can last for several months and even years (**Christian, 2015**).

11

COVID-19 & Haqua Revitalize® Therapy (HART)

IV.3. C- REACTIVE PROTEIN

IV.3.1. C-reactive protein and inflammation

Since inflammation is believed to have a role in the pathogenesis of cardiovascular events, measurement of markers of inflammation has been proposed as a method to improve the prediction of the risk of these events (**Paul et al., 2000**).

In the presence of an acute-phase stimulus, several proteins are up-regulated. C-reactive protein (CRP) is one of the most important acute-phase proteins. Stimuli that induce an acute-phase reaction can be of various origins: infectious (bacterial, fungal, mycobacterial, or severe viral), inflammatory, stress, tissue necrosis, trauma, childbirth, and neoplasia (**Séverine, 2004**).

11

COVID-19 & Haqua Revitalize® Therapy (HART)

IV.3.2. definition

C- reactive protein (CRP) is a major acute-phase plasma protein displaying rapid and pronounced rise of its serum concentration in response to infection or tissue injury **(Volanakis, 2001)**. CRP was so named because it was first discovered as a substance in the serum of patients with acute inflammation that reacted with the C- (capsular) polysaccharide of pneumococcus **(Moneer et al, 2012)**. C-reactive protein (CRP) is known to most clinicians as a marker of inflammation but has many other functions besides this **(Séverine et al., 2004)**.

11

COVID-19 & Haqua Revitalize® Therapy (HART)

IV.3.3. structure of the C-reactive protein

C-reactive protein (CRP) belongs to the pentraxin family of calcium dependent ligand-binding plasma proteins. The human CRP molecule is composed of five identical non-glycosylated polypeptide subunits each containing 206 amino acid residues. The protomers are non-covalently associated in an annular configuration with cyclic pentameric symmetry. The pentraxin family, named for its electron micrographic appearance from the Greek penta (five) ragos (berries), is highly conserved in evolution **(Amit et al., 2014)** (Figure05).

11

COVID-19 & Haqua Revitalize® Therapy (HART)

IV.3.4.Function of the C-reactive protein

The main biologic function of CRP is determined by its ability to recognize pathogens and damaged cells of the host and to mediate their elimination by recruiting the complement system and phagocytic cells (Volanakis, 2001) and (Séverine et al., 2004). CRP therefore is an important molecule in the host's innate immune system and in the protection against autoimmunity (Séverine et al., 2004).

IV.3.5.C-reactive protein level and clinical implication and indication

CRP usually isn't present in the blood. In adults, results may be reported as less than 0.8 mg/dl (less than 8 mg/l). An elvated CRP level may be present in rheumatoid artirits, rheumatic fever, complications of diabetes, obesity, cancer, acute bactérials and viral infections, inflammatory bowel disease, hodshkin's disease, and systemic lupus erytheromatosus (Lippincott and Wilkins, 2009).

11

COVID-19 & Haqua Revitalize® Therapy (HART)

VII. HOT WATER

VII.1. Definition of water

Water is the most important chemical component on the earth's surface (Garrette and Grisham, 2000). It is a unique, ubiquitous substance that is a major component of all living things (Kim and Johnson, 2001). It about 70% of Earth's surface, makes up about 70% of your mass, and is essential for life. Water is the only substance that exists naturally on Earth in all three physical states of matter: gas, liquid, and solid and it is always on the move among them (Shakhashiri, 2011).

11

COVID-19 & Haqua Revitalize® Therapy (HART)

Figure 13: Water molecules **(Shakhashiri, 2011)**

VII.4. Hydrotherapy

The use of water for various treatments (hydrotherapy) is probably as old as mankind. Hydrotherapy is one of the basic methods of treatment widely used in the system of natural medicine, which is also called as water therapy. Hydrotherapy is the external or internal use of water in any of its forms (water, ice, steam) for health promotion or treatment of various diseases with various temperatures, pressure, duration, and site. It is one of the naturopathic treatment modality used widely in ancient cultures including India, Egypt, and China **(Mooventhan et al., 2014).**

11

COVID-19 & Haqua Revitalize® Therapy (HART)

VII.5. The miracle and wonder of treatment with hot water

Heat is the only element that destroy harmful bacteria, melts the fats and neutrelizes the toxines that spread in our bodies from the food preservative today's world.

The only means to split H with O by heating water which will there after burn the O from water in a form of odoerless and colorless, however, drinking at least (8) glasses of hot water daily , with enough heat affordable for our bodies. We end up inhaling a large quantité of H, wich considered as the main body's nutrient element **(Alhajari, 2010).** ▶ Correction (AlHajri, 2010)

11, 13

COVID-19 & Haqua Revitalize® Therapy (HART)

VII.6. Benefits of drinking hot water

Prevent various diseases, symptoms and allergies. Heal people in pain, with sickness, allergies and diseases even if how critical it is. Get rid of fat. Reduce obesity, heals bronchial asthma, diabetes, hypertension, high cholesterol... etc, Improve brain memory. Possess a good looking body. To be healthy, we must drink the required quantity of Hot Water in a day. Health is wealth, so we have to keep a healthy body to have a wealthy lifestyle (**Alhadjri, 2010**) (Figure14). ▶ Correction (AlHajri, 2010)

11, 13

COVID-19 & Haqua Revitalize® Therapy (HART)
Materials and Methods

1. Materials

1.1. Animals

The experiment was performed on 20 males young rats Wistar Albinos, (1-2 Months) weighing between (57.1g-126.7g). All animals were born in animal house (university des frères Mentouri constantine), and they were housed in cages with free access to water and diet every day at room temperature. Composition of diet is shown at (Table 02).

1.2. Blood samples

After 21 days of experiment, animals were fasted overnight and the blood was obtained from the retro orbital sinus and collected into EDTA tubes.

11

COVID-19 & Haqua Revitalize® Therapy (HART)

2. Methods

2.1. Biochemical analysis

2.1. a. Treatment of rats

After acclimatization to the laboratory conditions for 10 days, the twenty rats were divided into four groups and fed for 21 days with control and experimental diets (table 03).

All animals in the groups I (C) and IV (HW) were fed with animal diets however the groups II (CH/W) and III (CH/HW) were fed with diet rich in trans fats, the groups I and II have drink normal water but III and IV have drink hot water (around 50°C) (table 10), the animals were kept in cages, the weight and diet and water consumed by rats were taken throughout the experiment at the same time. After 21days, the animals were fasted overnight, and the blood was collected for biochemical analysis.

11

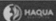

COVID-19 & Haqua Revitalize® Therapy (HART)

Table 03: Treatment of rats for 21 days

Experimental group	Treatment	Number of animals	Duration of experiment	Daily dose
GI(C)	Normal water +Animal Diet	5	21	175ml/5rats
GII(CH/W)	Normal water +Animal diet+Trans fats	5	21	175ml + 34g/5rats
GIII(CH/HW)	Hot water + Animal diet+Trans fats	5	21	175ml + 34g/5rats
GIV(HW)	Hot water+ Animal Diet	5	21	175ml/5rats

11

COVID-19 & Haqua Revitalize® Therapy (HART)

2.2. Histological analysis

After blood samples collection, the animals were kept in the laboratory for another extra 5 days of treatment, the G I (C) and G IV (HW) were fed with animal diet and supplemented with bread and they have drink normal water and hot water respectively, however the groups II and III they were fed with diet rich in trans fats and supplemented with animal fats which is source of saturated fatty acids and bread and they have drink normal and hot water respectively (Table04).

11

 HAQUA

COVID-19 & Haqua Revitalize® Therapy (HART)
Results and Discussions

1. Results

1.1. Animals investigations

1.1.1. Diet variation

- **Control group I (group C)**

The diet taken from the group I (C) during the first, second and third week was (46,71g±1.82), (59,03g±6.56) and (42,63g±9.51) respectively. There is a difference very highly significantly in diet consumption between weeks p= 0.002.

The tukey's test indicated that the diet consumed by rats in the second week is increased significantly when it is compared to the first week p=0.023. However the diet consumed by rats in the third week is decrease highly significantly when it is compared to the second week p=0.002 (Figure15) and (Table05 annex).

11

 HAQUA

COVID-19 & Haqua Revitalize® Therapy (HART)

- **Cholesterol/water group II (CH/W)**

  In the group II (CH/W), the consumption of diet during the first until the third week was (47.16g±5.39), (41.91g±2.19) and (43.32g±22.14) respectively. There is a difference in diet consumption between weeks p=0.806.

  The tukey's test indicated that the diet consumed by rats in the third week is decreased not significantly when compared to the first week p>0.05 (Figure 15) and (Table06 annex).

- **Cholesterol/hot water group III (group CH/HW)**

  The diet taken from the rats in group III (CH/HW) during three weeks was (49.71g±12.94), (22.30g±3.34) and (29.22g±20.16) respectively. There is a difference in diet consumption between weeks p=0.014.

  The tukey's test indicated that the diet consumed by rats in the second week is decreased significantly when it is compared to the first week p=0.013 (Figure15) and (Table07 annex).   11

COVID-19 & Haqua Revitalize® Therapy (HART)

- **Hot water group IV (group HW)**

  The diet taken from rats in group IV (HW) during the three weeks was (43.64g±5.12), (45.26g±13.06) and (33.99g±12.32) respectively. There is a difference in diet consumption between weeks p= 0.229.

  The tukey's test indicated that the diet consumed by rats in the third week is decrease not significantly when it is compared to the first week p>0.05 (Figure15) and (Table08 annex).

  11

COVID-19 & Haqua Revitalize® Therapy (HART)

1.1.2. The weight variation

- **Control group I (group C)**

The weight of rats group I (C) during the first, second and third weeks was (103,02g±1, 22), (101.15g±1.80) and (105.09g±2) respectively. There is a difference very highly significantly in weight values between groups of weeks p=0.003.

The tukey's test indicated that the weight of rats in the third week is increased significantly when it is compared to the second week p=0.002 (Figure16) and (table 05 annex).

- **Cholesterol/water group II (group CH/W)**

The weight of rats group (CH/W) during the first, second and the third weeks was (104,36g±3,59), (114,9g±5,59) and (127,88g±1,43) respectively. There is a difference very highly significantly in weight values betweens weeks p=0.000.

The tukey's test indicated that the weight of rats in the second week is increased highly significantly when it is compared to the first week p=0.001,and also in the third week is increased highly significantly when it is compared to the first and the second weeks p=0.000 (Figure16) and (Table 06 annex).

11

COVID-19 & Haqua Revitalize® Therapy (HART)

- **Cholesterol/hot water group III (group CH/HW)**

The weight of rats group (CH/HW) during the first, second and the third weeks was (69,29g±2.48), (79,11g±3.22) and (88,4g±2,15) respectively. There is a difference very highly significantly in weight values between weeks p=0.000.

The tukey's test indicated that the weight of rats in the second and the third weeks is increased very highly significantly when it is compared to the first week p=0.000, and in the third week is increased very highly significantly when it is compared to the second week p=0.000 (Figure16) and (Table 07annex).

- **Hot water group IV (group HW)**

The weight of rats group (HW) during the first, second and the third weeks was (74,86g±1,56) (66,15g±2.20) and (73,38g±3,18) respectively. There is a difference very highly significantly in weight values between weeks p=0.000.

The tukey's test indicated that the weight of rats in the second week is decreased very highly significantly when it is compared to the first week p= 0.000 and in the third week is increased when it is compared to the second week p=0.000 (Figure16) (Table 08annex).

11

COVID-19 & Haqua Revitalize® Therapy (HART)

1.2.1. Lipids status

1.2.1. a. Total cholesterol

The concentration of total cholesterol was (0.73g±0.10) in group I,(0.81g±0.14) in group II, (0.80g±0.03) in group III and (0.89g±0.10) in group IV, our data indicated that the cholesterol is decreased in group III when it is compared to the group II and IV but not significantly p>0.05 (figure 18).

1.2.1. b. Triglyceride

The concentration of Triglyceride was (0.54g±0.11) in group I, (0.57g±0.17) in group II , (0.44g±0.09) in group III and (0.77g±0.25) in group IV. The Triglyceride concentration was decreased in group III but not significantly when it is compared to the other groups p>0.05 (Figure 19).

11

COVID-19 & Haqua Revitalize® Therapy (HART)

1.2.1. c. HDL-c

The concentration of HDL-c was in group I (0.73g±0.11), in group II (0.79g+0.15), in the group III (0.81g±0.07), and in group IV (0.84g+0.17). We have observed an increase in the concentration of HDL-c in group III when it is compared to the group I and II, however the concentration of HDL-c in the group IV was higher than the other group but not significantly p>0.05 (Figure 20).

1.2.1. d. LDL-c

The results of the determination of LDL-c in group I (0.08g±0.01), group II (0.13g±0.06), group III (0.10g±0.03) and group IV (0.10g+0.02) showed that there was a difference between groups but not significantly p>0.05 Our data indicated that the LDL-c concentration was decreased in group III and IV treated with hot water when it is compared to the other groups treated with normal water p>0.05 (Figure21).

1.2.2. hs-CRP

The values of hs-CRP were in the group I (0.27g±0.12), group II (0.66g+0.28), group III (0.37g+0.12) and group IV (0.7g+0.18). Our result indicated that the hs-CRP concentration was decreased in group III when it is compared to the groups II and IV but it was slightly higher than group I (Figure22).

11

COVID-19 & Haqua Revitalize® Therapy (HART)

1.3. Behavior and morphological investigations

During our study we have noticed that the animals in the group III (CH/HW) are very active when it is compared to other groups. Also we have observed nodules(0.47g, 1.50g and 3.77g) in the neck of three rats in group II (CH/W) and more adipose tissue , otherwise the other groups don't present any nodules and less adipose tissue (photo 01) also we have observed modification on renal color in rat at group II (photo 02).

1.4. Histological investigation

The weight of organs (liver, heart, aorta, spleen and intestine) in group I was (5.69g, 0.46g, 0.15g,0.51g and 11.65g) respectively. The weight of organs (liver, heart, aorta, spleen and intestine) in group II was (6.14g, 0.55g, 0.17g, 0.64g and 9.79g) respectively. The weight of organs (liver, heart, aorta, spleen and intestine) in group III was (4.70g, 0.40g, 0.15g and 9.33g) respectively. The weight of organs (liver, heart, aorta, spleen and intestine) in group IV was (5.50g, 0.42g, 0.15g and 0.40g) respectively (Figure 27). The organs fixed into the formal solution are kept for future work. 11

COVID-19 & Haqua Revitalize® Therapy (HART)

Discussion

We could explain that by the influence of hot water on the enzymes which helps the metabolism reaction (**Alhajri, 2010**).

Our results are in agreement with those of (**Alhadjri, 2010**) who reported that hot water

► Correction (AlHajri, 2010)

dissolve the lipids in our organism and healing the inflammation. 11

COVID-19 & Haqua Revitalize® Therapy (HART)
Conclusion

The recommended consumption of hot water play a role on the body weight, and it has an anti-inflammatory effect for long or short term. So the use of hot water seems to have an interest in prevention of atherosclerosis and inflammatory bowel disease (IBD).

The present experimental finding showed that hot water therapy process has a positive effect on the inflammation and a decrease in lipids status.

Based on the present results, our futur work and prespectives can evaluate many topics:

-We need to keep the water at the same temperature (50°C) for the hole day and night.   11

 HAQUA   © Copyright – All Rights Reserved – Faris AlHajri-Haqua Wellness

COVID-19 & Haqua Revitalize® Therapy (HART)
Reference (part)

-Aaron S B and Andrew P. (2015). The Role of Vitamin D in Inflammatory Bowel Disease. Healthcare. (3): 338-350.

-Alberti S., Schuster G., Parini P., Feltkamp D., Diczfalusy U., Rudling M., Angelin B., Björkhem I., Pettersson S., Gustafsson J. (2001). Hepatic cholesterol metabolism and resistance to dietary cholesterol in LXR beta-deficient mice. The Journal of Clinical Investigation. 107(4): 565–573.

-Aldons J L. (2000). Atherosclerosis. Nature. 407(6801): 233–241.

-Alhajri F. (2010). The miracle & wonders of treatment from hot water: hot water miracles. 1-108.
11

 HAQUA   © Copyright – All Rights Reserved – Faris AlHajri-Haqua Wellness

COVID-19 & Haqua Revitalize® Therapy (HART)
Summary

In the present study, we evaluated the benefit of hot water therapy on the inflammation induced by saturated and Trans fats during 21 days in rats, which was evaluated using the detection of hs-CRP and lipids status.

The results showed that the amount of hot water 60-175ml per day for rats could decrease the levels of hs-CRP and lipids status (T-Ch, TG and LDL-c) and increase the concentration of HDL-c.

For this reason, we considered that the hot water is a natural hydrotherapy during short or long term dependent on type of disease.

11

 HAQUA

COVID-19 & Haqua Revitalize® Therapy (HART)
Benefits of Drinking Hot Water

Therapeutic Methods of Drinking Hot Water (TMDHW) - For Adults

* The recommended consumption of Hot Water shall be at 3 liters daily minimum up to 4 liters maximum.

*Glass, mug or tumbler size - 500 ml, taken in different gulps, not one gulp.

* The maximum consumption of Hot Water shall be 1 liter within One Hour.

11, 13

 HAQUA

COVID-19 & Haqua Revitalize® Therapy (HART)
Option I – Drinking Method for glass size 500 ml

* One to two glasses early in the morning, once you wake up and before brushing your teeth – at standing position (Very important)

* One glass, after brushing your teeth, before having your breakfast.

*One to two glasses throughout the morning.

*One glass 15-30 minutes before lunch. (Very important).

*One to two glasses in the evening.

* One glass, one hour before going to bed (optional.)   11, 13

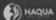 HAQUA   © Copyright – All Rights Reserved – Faris AlHajri-Haqua Wellness

COVID-19 & Haqua Revitalize® Therapy (HART)
Option 2 – Drinking Method for glass size 240-300 ml

* Two glasses of hot water, early in the morning, once you wake up and before brushing your teeth – at standing position - Very important

*One glass of hot water, after brushing your teeth, before having your breakfast (optional).

*Two to three glasses of hot water throughout the morning.

* One glass of hot water at least 15-30 minutes before lunch – Very important.

*Two to three glasses of hot water throughout the evening.

*One glass of hot water, one hour before going to bed.

- The temperature of water shall be around 50oC (122oF), a little bit less than the temperature of hot tea (Alhadjri, 2010).   ► Correction (AlHajri, 2010)   11, 13

 HAQUA   © Copyright – All Rights Reserved – Faris AlHajri-Haqua Wellness

COVID-19 & Haqua Revitalize® Therapy (HART)

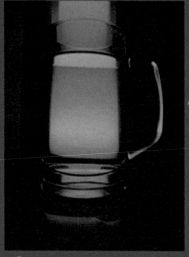

Why Haqua
(Hot Water)?

COVID-19 & Haqua Revitalize® Therapy (HART)

Haqua Revitalize® Therapy w.r.t. Humans' Cosmic Life

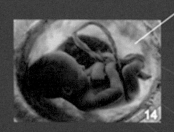

Amniotic Fluid/Amnii

99% Water   15

37.5°C (99.5°F)   16

Hot Water

Source of Creation & Growth

14

COVID-19 & Haqua Revitalize® Therapy (HART)

3 Basic Functions of Haqua Revitalize® Therapy

1. Kills Harmful Bacteria

2. Melts the Fat Deposits (Lipids)

3. Neutralizes Toxins

In 1877, two researchers, Downes & Blunt, discovered that sunlight can destroy harmful bacteria. Without sunlight, you could not remain alive an hour.　**17**

 HAQUA

COVID-19 & Haqua Revitalize® Therapy (HART)

Water – Human Body

Lungs-90%	Blood-82%
Brain-76%	Muscles-75%
Bones-25%	Body-75%

"You're not sick; you're thirsty. Don't treat thirst with medication" ~Dr. F. Batmanghelidj[18]

 HAQUA

COVID-19 & Haqua Revitalize® Therapy (HART)

Oxygen w.r.t. Haqua Revitalize® Therapy

Blood Oxygen Levels-Lungs- 95-100% [19]	**Brain-20%** [19]
RBC (Hemoglobin) - Blood [20]	**Atmosphere- 21%**

Body's Mass- 65% [21]

HART-100%

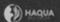

COVID-19 & Haqua Revitalize® Therapy (HART)

Hydrogen w.r.t. Haqua Revitalize® Therapy

$$O_2 + Energy + 2H_2 = 2H_2O$$
(Antoine Lavoisier-1783) [22]

Conversely !

$$2H_2O + Energy = O_2 + 2H_2$$

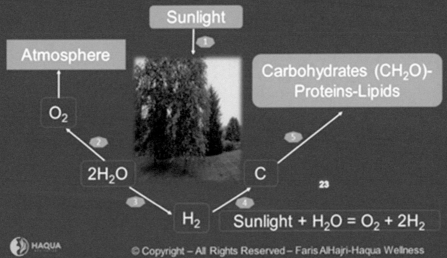

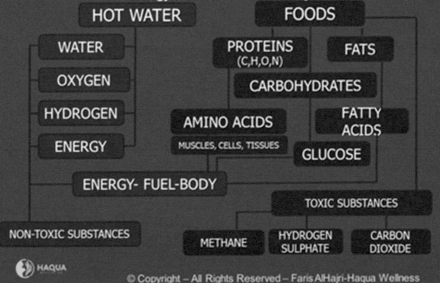

COVID-19 & Haqua Revitalize® Therapy (HART)

**Exceptional Therapeutic Methods of Haqua Gulping (TMHG)
for Prevention & dealing with COVID-19 (Adults)**

- **1st Day (In Full Isolation)**

1. **Drink a glass/mug/tumbler of 500 ml/17 oz up to one liter/34 oz of Hot Water (Haqua) at 1-2 hours intervals —** highly advised to reach five liters (169 oz) at 50ºC/122º F within the first 24 hours.

2. **Full Hot Water Fasting — Refrain completely from eating or drinking anything besides hot water as mentioned in (1) above.**

3. **Apply both Haqua Compress Method (HCM) and Haqua Steam Method (HSM) every time whenever possible, as recommended (►See Sections 3 and 4)**

4. **Abide your physician's instructions (medical doctor), strictly follow and his/her advice.**

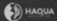 HAQUA

COVID-19 & Haqua Revitalize® Therapy (HART)

**Exceptional Therapeutic Methods of Haqua Gulping (TMHG)
for Prevention & dealing with COVID-19 (Adults)**

- **2nd and 3rd Days (In Full Isolation)**

1. **Drink a glass/mug/tumbler of 500 ml/17 oz up to one liter/34 oz of Hot Water (Haqua) at two-hour intervals — highly advised between 3-4 liters/101-135 oz at 50º C/122º F.**

2. **Full Liquid Diet — No solid foods at all, and only consume liquids such as hot soups, besides hot water as mentioned in (1) above.**

3. **Apply both Haqua Compress Method (HCM) and Haqua Steam Method (HSM) every time whenever possible, as recommended (►See Sections 3 and 4).**

4. **Abide by your physician's instructions (medical doctor): strictly follow his/her advice.**

 HAQUA

COVID-19 & Haqua Revitalize® Therapy (HART)

Exceptional Therapeutic Methods of Haqua Gulping (TMHG) for Prevention & dealing with COVID-19 (Adults)

• **4th Day through 2 weeks, or until recovery (In Full Isolation)**

1. **Drink a glass/mug/tumbler of 500 ml/17 oz up to one liter/34 oz of Hot Water (Haqua) at two hour intervals — highly advised between 3-4 liters/101-135 oz at 50° C/122° F.**

2. **Half Liquid Diet — Limit solid foods and consume liquids, such as hot soups, besides hot water as mentioned in (1) above on the second day.**

3. **Apply both Haqua Compress Method (HCM) and Haqua Steam Method (HSM) every time whenever possible, as recommended (▶See Sections 3 and 4).**

4. **Abide by your physician's instructions (medical doctor): strictly follow his/her advice.**

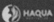

COVID-19 & Haqua Revitalize® Therapy (HART)

Exceptional Therapeutic Methods of Haqua Gulping (TMHG) for Prevention & dealing with COVID-19 (Adults)

• **After 2 weeks (until fully recovered)**

1. **Follow the Therapeutic Methods of Haqua Gulping (TMHG) on regular basis as recommended (▶See Section 5).**

2. **Full Liquid Diet — No solid foods and only consume liquids, such as hot soups, besides hot water as mentioned in (1) above.**

3. **Apply both Haqua Compress Method (HCM) and Haqua Steam Method (HSM) every time whenever possible, as recommended (▶See Sections 3 and 4).**

4. **Abide by your physician's instructions (medical doctor): strictly follow his/her advice.**

COVID-19 & Haqua Revitalize® Therapy (HART)

Therapeutic Methods of Haqua Gulping (TMHG)

Haqua Common Gulping Method (HCGM)

[glass size 500ml/17 oz] - For Adults

1. One glass upon waking and on a 'clean' mouth* – at a standing position.*
2. One glass between 7:00-10:00 a.m.
3. One glass 15-30 minutes before lunch.**
4. One glass between 2:00-4:00 p.m.
5. One glass in the evening, 15-30 minutes before dinner.**
6. One glass an hour before sleep.**

 HAQUA

COVID-19 & Haqua Revitalize® Therapy (HART)

1. Notes:
2. *Haqua should be taken before brushing teeth, mouthwash, or eating anything.
3. ** Should be given high consideration. Haqua will detoxify the body, removing toxins which are in the form of gases (Carbon Dioxide-CO22, Hydrogen Sulfide-H2S, Nitrogen-N, and Methane-CH4).

COVID-19 & Haqua Revitalize® Therapy (HART)

Therapeutic Methods of Haqua Gulping (TMHG)

Haqua Common Gulping Method (HCGM) – [glass size 500ml/17 oz] - For Adults

1. The daily recommended consumption of Haqua (Hot Water) is a minimum of 3 liters/101oz and maximum of 4 liters/135oz.

2. The water volume taken should not exceed 500ml/17oz at one time, and a maximum of one liter in the span of an hour.

3. The recommended temperature of Haqua is fixed at around 50ºC (122ºF), a little bit less than the temperature of hot tea or hot coffee.

COVID-19 & Haqua Revitalize® Therapy (HART)

Haqua Compress Method (HCM)

Option I (recommended)

• Boil water in a wireless water boiler and place it in a safe area near your shower.

• Take a hot shower and thoroughly clean your body.

• After showering, pour hot water from the shower tap into a container or basin, filling only ¾ of the container.

• Add boiled water from the water boiler to the container or basin.

• Immerse a small towel (approximately 30cmx30cm/1ftx1ft in size) halfway or fully in the basin filled with Haqua (hot water). Maintain a temperature of around 70ºC-80ºC/160ºF-180ºF in the basin.

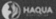

COVID-19 & Haqua Revitalize® Therapy (HART)

Haqua Compress Method (HCM)

Option I (cont'd)

- Test the temperature of the wet towel with your hand. Make sure that it is not too hot.

- Gently rub and massage all parts of your body, following the Therapeutic Steps below. Each part should be done once or twice. After each step, re-wet your towel. This will maintain a steady heat throughout the process.

- The overall process should take around four minutes.

- It is recommended to use this therapy once daily, four to five days per week.

- Two towels will be needed.

COVID-19 & Haqua Revitalize® Therapy (HART)

Haqua Compress Method (HCM)

Therapeutic Steps: Towel 1

- Face.

- Neck.

- Right shoulder, covering the front and back parts of your shoulder.

- Left shoulder, covering the front and back parts of your shoulder.

- Right hand up to the fingers.

- Left hand up to the fingers.

- Chest down to the stomach.

COVID-19 & Haqua Revitalize® Therapy (HART)
Haqua Compress Method (HCM)

Therapeutic Steps: Towel 1 (cont'd)
- Right leg down to the ankle.
- Left leg down to the ankle.
- Right foot, covering the tops and bottoms of the foot and toes.
- Left foot, covering the tops and bottoms of the foot and toes.

Therapeutic Steps: Towel 2
- Apply to the genital part of your body.

COVID-19 & Haqua Revitalize® Therapy (HART)
Haqua Compress Method (HCM)

Option II
- Take a hot shower and thoroughly clean your body.
- Using a small towel (approximately 30cmx30cm/1ftx1ft in size), increase the temperature of the water. As the hot water continues to run, gently rub your body, following the steps mentioned below.
- The Haqua Compress Method is recommended to be performed by a professional Holistic Health Therapist or Massage Therapist in this field to prevent injury.

COVID-19 & Haqua Revitalize® Therapy (HART)

Haqua Steam Method (HSM)

Therapeutic Methods for personal or home use

- Fill one third of an electric water boiler with clean tap water and cover as much of the body as possible with a blanket or towel.
- Boil the water and keep the cover of the electric boiler opened.
- Keep the steam at a temperature that does not burn your face.
- Inhale the steam with your mouth and release it through the nose. Then inhale with your nose and release through your mouth.

COVID-19 & Haqua Revitalize® Therapy (HART)
Haqua Steam Method (HSM)- Cont'd

Therapeutic Methods for personal or home use (cont'd)

- Inhale from one side of your nose and release the steam through the other side of your nose, and vice versa.
- Use this method for around 4 minutes.
- The Haqua Steam Method is recommended to be performed by a professional Holistic Health Therapist or Massage Therapist in this field to prevent injury.

COVID-19 & Haqua Revitalize® Therapy (HART)
Benefits of Hydrogen in Human Body

The mole fraction for water is 67% hydrogen and 33% oxygen. [24]

Albert Szent-Györgyi, a 1937 Biologist and Nobel Prize winner, was the first to prove that the human body stores hydrogen in many of its organs. He referred to this as 'hydrogen pooling' and he identified the organs that pool the greatest amounts of hydrogen. [25]

 HAQUA

COVID-19 & Haqua Revitalize® Therapy (HART)
Benefits of Hydrogen in Human Body

The hydrogen atom is the smallest of all the elements and has as much antioxidant power as any of the larger, complex compounds. [26]

Szent-Györgyi said in his 1937 Nobel lecture: "A living cell requires energy not only for all its functions, but also for the maintenance of its structure… [this brings] out the fact that our body really only knows one fuel, hydrogen." Without energy, life would be instantly extinguished, and the cellular fabric would collapse. [27]

 HAQUA

COVID-19 & Haqua Revitalize® Therapy (HART)

Free-radical Damage
Hydrogen Depletion

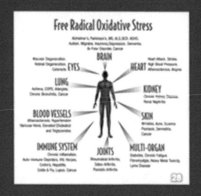

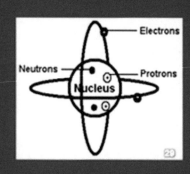

COVID-19 & Haqua Revitalize® Therapy (HART)

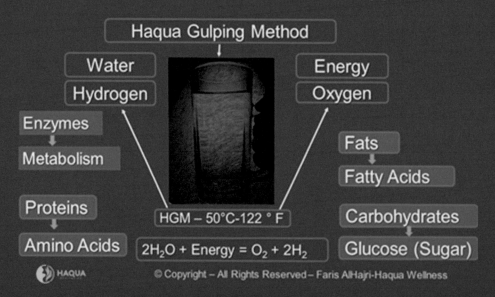

COVID-19 & Haqua Revitalize® Therapy (HART)
Benefits of Energy In Human Body

Thermogenesis is a generation or production of heat, especially by physiological processes. [30]

Thermal convection is the transfer of energy between an object and its environment, due to fluid motion. The human body must maintain a consistent internal temperature in order to maintain healthy bodily functions. [31]

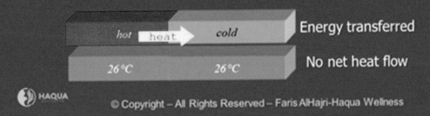

Energy transferred

No net heat flow

COVID-19 & Haqua Revitalize® Therapy (HART)
Energy Transfer in Human Body

The Second Law of Thermodynamics (first expression): Heat transfer occurs spontaneously from higher- to lower-temperature bodies, but never spontaneously in the reverse direction. [32]

Convection is the process by which heat is transferred by movement of a heated fluid, such as air or water. [33]

COVID-19 & Haqua Revitalize® Therapy (HART)

Energy Transfer in the Human Body

If you add heat to a system, there are only two things that can be done: change the internal energy of the system or cause the system to do work (or, of course, some combination of the two). [34]

Hot Water: 50ºC-122ºF

Body's Temperature: 37ºC-98.6ºF

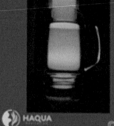

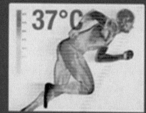

COVID-19 & Haqua Revitalize® Therapy (HART)

Calorie (cal) = Thermal Energy

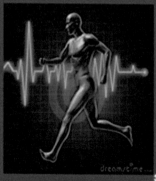

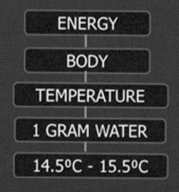

ENERGY

BODY

TEMPERATURE

1 GRAM WATER

14.5ºC - 15.5ºC

References

1. Coronavirus Infections. MedlinePlus. U.S. National Library of Medicine. https://medlineplus.gov/coronavirusinfections.html - accessed February 28, 2020.

2. "Operations Dashboard for ArcGIS". gisanddata.maps.arcgis.com. The Center for Systems Science and Engineering (CSSE) is a research collective housed within the Department of Civil and Systems Engineering (CaSE) at Johns Hopkins University (JHU). 28 January 2020. Archived from the original on 28 January 2020. Retrieved 3 February 2020.

3. "Coronavirus Toll Update: Cases & Deaths by Country of Wuhan, China Virus - Worldometer". www.worldometers.info. Archived from the original on 2 February 2020. Retrieved 2 February 2020.

4. Coronavirus. Wikipedia the free encyclopedia. https://en.wikipedia.org/wiki/Coronavirus - accessed February 28, 2020.

5. About Coronavirus Disease 2019 (COVID-19). Minnesota Department of Health. https://www.health.state.mn.us/diseases/coronavirus/basics.html - accessed February 28, 2020.

6. How COVID-19 Kills: The New Coronavirus Disease Can Take A Deadly Turn. NPR Radio. Maria Godoy. February 14, 2020. Weekend Edition Sunday. https://www.npr.org/sections/goatsandsoda/2020/02/14/805289669/how-covid-19-kills-the-new-coronavirus-disease-can-take-a-deadly-turn - accessed February 28, 2020.

7. Fighting Against Coronavirus. Research Products for COVID-19 (SARS-CoV-2). RayBiotech. https://www.raybiotech.com/coronavirus-research-products-sars-cov-2-covid-19/ - accessed February 28, 2020.

8. Zhang JM, An J. Cytokines, inflammation, and pain. Int Anesthesiol Clin. 2007 Spring;45(2):27-37. doi: 10.1097/AIA.0b013e318034194e. PMID: 17426506; PMCID: PMC2785020.- https://www.ncbi.nlm.nih.gov/pmc/articles/PMC2785020/ - accessed March 01, 2020

9. Here's What Happens to the Body After Contracting the Coronavirus. Shawn Radcliffe. February 20, 2020. https://www.healthline.com/health-news/heres-what-happens-to-the-body-after-contracting-the-coronavirus - accessed February 28, 2020.

10. Tenets of Osteopathic Medicine. American osteopathic Association. https://osteopathic.org/about/leadership/aoa-governance-documents/tenets-of-osteopathic-medicine/ - accessed February 28, 2020.

11. AlHajri Faris. (2010). The miracle & wonders of treatment from hot water: hot water miracles. 1-108. https://www.farisalhajri.com

12. The effects of hot water on inflammation induced by hypercholesterolemia in rats. University of Frères Mentouri Constantine. Ministry of Higher Education and Scientific Research. Guennoub S, Redouane R, Dr Messoudi s, Pr Zerizer S, Dr Aribi B. http://fac.umc.edu.dz/snv/faculte/biblio/mmf/2017/The%20Effect%20of%20hot%20water%20on%20inflammation%20induced%20by%20hypercholesterolemia%20in%20rats.pdf - accessed February 28, 2020.

13. Faris AlHajri-Ph.D.(A.M.). The Miracle & Wonders of Treatment from Hot Water - Hot Water Miracles by Faris Alhajri. https://www.authorhouse.com/BookStore/BookDetails/290003-The-Miracle-Wonders-of-Treatment-from-Hot-Water. https://www.farisalhajri.com. https://www.haquawellness.com

14. Image: http://www.online-sciences.com/wp-content/uploads/2016/05/placenta-importance-in-fetal-development-8-300x200.jpg

15. Kaldas Center for Fertility, & Surgery Pregnancy, SC. http://kaldascenter.com/resources/second-trimester/ - accessed May 1, 2016.

16. The Fetal Life-Support System: Placenta, Umbilical Cord, & Amniotic Sac, American Pregnancy Association. http://americanpregnancy.org/while-pregnant/fetal-life-support-system/ - accessed May 1, 2016.

17. Section 0 – Principles of Health. Second Law of Health – Sunlight. THE SUNLIGHT ON YOUR BODY. Part 4b. http://www.pathlights.com/nr encyclopedia/00prin4b.htm - accessed May 21, 2008- updated 19 December 2012

18. "You're not sick; you're thirsty. Don't treat thirst with medication.", The Water Cure, Dr. F. Batmanghelidj, http://www.watercure.com/ - accessed 17 May 2008

19. Hypoxemia (low blood oxygen). Mayo Clinic. https://www.mayoclinic.org/symptoms/hypoxemia/basics/definition/sym-20050930 - accessed June 1, 2016.

20. Oxygen Saturation. Wikipedia. The free Encyclopedia. https://en.wikipedia.org/wiki/Oxygen saturation (medicine) – accessed June 1, 2016.

21. Composition of the human body. Wikipedia the free encyclopedia. https://en.wikipedia.org/wiki/Composition of the human body - accessed June 2, 2016.

22. Hydrogen. Wikipedia. The Free Encyclopedia. http://en.wikipedia.org/wiki/Hydrogen - accessed June 6, 2009.

23. Hydrogen… Longevity's Missing Link. Patrick Flanagan MD. Nexus December, 1994 – January 1995. http://www.whale.to/a/flanagan.html - accessed May 15, 2016.

24. Percent Composition. Robert Belford, Professor (Chemistry) at University of Arkansas at Little Rock. https://chem.libretexts.org/Courses University of Arkansas Little Rock/Chem 1402%3A General Chemistry 1 (Belford) Text/2%3A Atoms%2C Molecules%2C and Ions/2.10%3A Percent Composition – accessed March 02, 2020.

References (Cont'd.)

25. Dancing with water. Hydrogen: Fuel of Life. http://www.dancingwithwater.com/articles/hydrogen-fuel-of-life/ - accessed May 28, 2016.

26..Hydrogen & Oxygen THE ULTIMATE ANTIOXIDANT. Tuberose.com. http://www.tuberose.com/Hydrogen and Oxygen.html - accessed June 6, 2009.

27. 1071. A LBERT S ZEN T- GYÖRGY I. Oxidation, energy transfer, and vitamins. Nobel Lecture, December 11, 1937. http://www.nobelprize.org/nobel prizes/medicine/laureates/1937/szent-gyorgyi-lecture.pdf - accessed May 25, 2016.

28. http://www.geneactivatornrf2.org/what-is-oxidative-stress/

29. http://sciencedoing.blogspot.com/2012/09/free-radicals-cause-and-concern.html.

30. Thermogenesis. The Free Dictionary by Farlex. http://medical-dictionary.thefreedictionary.com/thermogenesis- accessed January 9, 2013.

31- Heat Transfer. Wikipedia the Free Encyclopedia. https://en.wikipedia.org/wiki/Heat transfer#cite ref-25 – accessed October 18, 2016.

32. INTRODUCTION TO THE SECOND LAW OF THERMODYNAMICS: HEAT ENGINES AND THEIR EFFICIENCY. https://opentextbc.ca/physicstestbook2/chapter/introduction-to-the-second-law-of-thermodynamics-heat-engines-and-their-efficiency/ - accessed March 01, 2020.

33. Convection. Encyclopaedia Britannica. https://www.britannica.com/science/convection - accessed March 01, 2020.

34. Laws of Thermodynamics. About education. http://physics.about.com/od/thermodynamics/a/lawthermo 3.htm - accessed December 9, 2012.

35. Image :https://www.pinterest.com/explore/human-body-temperature/

36. Image: http://physics.about.com/od/glossary/g/heat.htm

37. Heat Energy - Definition and Examples. about education. http://physics.about.com/od/glossary/g/heat.htm - accessed December 9, 2012.

Faris AlHajri – Ph.D. (A.M.)
Haqua Wellness
Haquawellness.com
Farisalhajri.com
Email- faris@farisalhajri.com

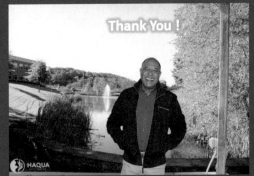

Credits!

Covers Designed by: Authorhouse

Copy editing and proof reading by: C. Klein

Formatted by : Authorhouse

About the Author

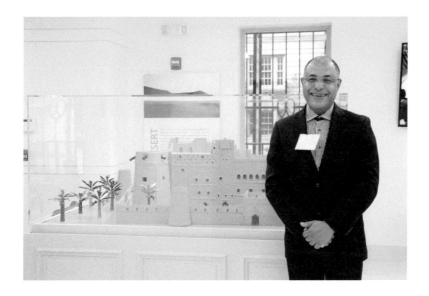

Faris AlHajri –Ph.D.(A.M.) is a certified Integrative Nutrition Health Coach from the Institute for Integrative Nutrition (IIN), New York, a Holistic Health & Wellness international renowned speaker and expert, entrepreneur, researcher, author of two books, discoverer of "Haqua Revitalize®" Therapy (HART), and president and founder of Haqua Wellness, Virginia, US.

He spoke at (8) International conferences as organizing committee member, speaker, chair, etc.; interviewed and featured in (92) international media, and conducted (65) lectures and seminars in Universities, Schools, Health Organizations, Mosques, Churches, and Public; in different countries worldwide; Melbourne (Australia), San Diego (Ca, US), UK, India, Philippines, Malaysia, Oman, Qatar, Saudi Arabia, and UAE

Faris is driven by a found desire to promote healthy living and has completely devoted his life to spread natural health and wellness awareness. An internationally travelled expert, conducting workshops and seminars. His ongoing goal is to help all individuals understand the importance of the miraculous benefits of HART. His Haqua Wellness office is located is located in Virginia Tech Corporate Research Center, Virginia, US. His main two strategies are to conduct clinical research studies in human subjects on the effectiveness of HART, and set up Haqua Wellness projects globally in various sizes to keep promoting his holistic health and wellness initiatives.

Printed in the United States
By Bookmasters